"Required reading for anyone truly interested in the role of meditation in the healing process."

—Arielle Ford, author of *Hot Chocolate for the Mystical Soul*

"Dharma Singh Khalsa shows us how the tremendous power of medical meditation can heal not only the body but also the mind and soul. I strongly recommend it."

—Deepak Chopra, M.D., author of *How to Know God*

"Activate and use your deep natural abilities now with Dr. Khalsa's book."

—Mark Victor Hansen, co-creator, #1 *New York Times* bestselling series of *Chicken Soup for the Soul*

"Within these very pages is the best knowledge you can find. Everybody must seek it out."

—Yogi Bhajan, Ph.D., Master of Kundalini and White Tantric Yoga

"Breathe deeply and listen to Dr.Dharma."

—*The Palm Beach Post*

PRAISE FOR
FOOD AS MEDICINE

"Provides a wealth of practical tips for living a long, healthy life. Dr. ʹalsa's extensive recommendations are well researched, concise, ., most important, easy to implement."

—Julian Whitaker, MD, Editor, *Health & Healing* magazine

ute, thought-provoking testimony to the veracity and wis-
ut alternative healing practices. It is a well-conceived, thorough
de for anyone seeking wellness through the wonderful medicinal power of food."

—Cary Neff, author of *Conscious Cuisine* and Executive Chef,
La Costa Resort and Spa

"On the cutting edge of dietary intelligence, a natural resource for healing, rich in wisdom, knowledge, and practical application. Highly recommended."

—Leanne Backer, chef and co-author of *The Chopra Cookbook:*
Nourishing Body and Soul

"While an insightful spiritual guide to eating, *Food as Medicine* also offers a bonanza of research-based nutritional pearls. It now holds a prominent place in my library."

— -David Leonardi, M.D., Medical Director, Cenegenics Medical Institute,
Las Vegas, NV

PRAISE FOR DHARMA SINGH KHALSA, M.D., AND HIS NATIONAL BESTSELLER *MEDITATION AS MEDICINE*

"Intelligent, accessible, and free of cant and hyperbole."
—*The Dallas Morning*

"Explores one of the most ancient methods of healing known to humankind, whose benefits have been affirmed by hundreds of careful scientific studies. . . . Whether you are a beginner in meditation or a veteran, you will benefit from this very wise book."
—Larry Dossey, M.D., author of *Reinventing Medicine* and *Healing Words*

"An extraordinary guide to tapping into the innate healing powers we all have. I highly recommend it to everyone at all levels."
—Judith Orloff, M.D., author of *Dr. Judith Orloff's Guide to Intuitive Healing*

FOOD
as
MEDICINE

How to Use Diet, Vitamins, Juices, and Herbs

For a Healthier, Happier, and Longer Life

DHARMA SINGH KHALSA, M.D.

ATRIA BOOKS

New York   London   Toronto   Sydney

This book is lovingly dedicated to
Yogi Bhajan and his wife, Bibiji Inderjit Kaur,
who were kind enough to share their vast knowledge
on using food as medicine.

Kundalini Research Institute

This Seal of Approval is granted only to those products which have been approved through the KRI Review process for accuracy and integrity of those portions which embody the technology of Kundalini Yoga and 3HO Lifestyle as taught by Yogi Bhajan.

The ideas, procedures, and suggestions in this book are not intended as a substitute for the medical advice of a trained health professional. All matters regarding your health require medical supervision. Consult your physician before adopting the suggestions in this book, as well as about any condition that may require diagnosis or medical attention. The author and publisher disclaim any liability arising directly or indirectly from the use of the book or of any products mentioned herein.

ATRIA BOOKS
1230 Avenue of the Americas
New York, NY 10020

Copyright © 2003 by Dharma Singh Khalsa, M.D.

All rights reserved, including the right to reproduce
this book or portions thereof in any form whatsoever.
For information address Atria Books, 1230 Avenue
of the Americas, New York, NY 10020

Library of Congress Cataloging-in-Publication Data is available.

ISBN-13: 978-0-7434-4226-8
ISBN-10:   0-7434-4226-1
ISBN-13: 978-0-7434-4228-2 (Pbk)
ISBN-10:   0-7434-4228-8 (Pbk)

First Atria Books trade paperback edition January 2004

10   9   8

ATRIA BOOKS is a trademark of Simon & Schuster, Inc.

Manufactured in the United States of America

For information regarding special discounts for bulk purchases, please contact
Simon & Schuster Special Sales at 1-800-456-6798 or business@simonandschuster.com.

CONTENTS

PART 2

Eat This for That

PART I

The Cutting Edge of Medicine

CHAPTER 1

Spiritual Nutrition

What a beautiful day for an epiphany. Here I am on a seventeen-mile mountain bike ride at an altitude of 6,700 feet in Jackson Hole, Wyoming. The air I'm breathing in this pristine environment is clear and cool. It's a fresh, warm, early summer afternoon, and along with some new friends I am relishing a bit of free time at one of the most enlightening medical conferences I've ever attended. The event is devoted to using food to prevent and heal illness, and I feel so inspired that I can't wait to get back to Tucson to begin writing. I want very much to share all this new and exciting information with you, such as

- how cancer can be prevented and reversed using food.
- how heart disease can be treated using specific foods and nutrients.
- how Alzheimer's disease can be prevented and treated with food and nutrients.
- how food can cure chronic fatigue.
- how diet and vitamins can restore emotional energy.

It turns out that every major ailment has a specific natural food prescription that can reverse its course. This is the cutting edge of medicine.

The Buddha wrote:

> Don't chase after the past,
> Don't seek the future.
> The past is gone.
> The future hasn't come yet.

See clearly on the spot
That object which is *now*.

In my work as a physician specializing in integrative medicine, I have used nutrition as part of my practice for many years. This type of medicine, as you may know, is the emerging field that blends the best of conventional Western science with ancient healing therapies such as yoga, meditation, nutrition, herbal medicines, and acupuncture. Because I use both Eastern and Western medicine, many of my patients have made unexpected recoveries from illnesses they had been struggling with for many years. Some of them have considered their recoveries to be miraculous, but I see only the natural outcome of good science and good sense. The one thing I have come to believe while participating in these recoveries with my patients—whom I call my healing partners—is that your body has the ability to heal itself if you just give it a chance. Using food as medicine gives my patients the greatest chance of all to heal.

One of the chief reasons my program has been so successful is that it treats each person as a unique being. If you come to see me, I take into consideration your biochemical uniqueness and then design a program to restore you to maximum physical, mental, emotional, and spiritual health. When that happens—when you once again attain a healing balance in your body, mind, and spirit—it certainly feels miraculous. It is the answer to your deepest prayer.

The practical use of modern nutritional principles, which I will present in this book, will allow you to activate your own natural inner healing force and bring you back into a balanced state. Since no two patients are alike, no two require exactly the same therapy. When a patient comes to me for pain, fatigue, memory loss, cancer recovery, high blood pressure, or some other ailment, I always have my nutritionist, Luz-Elena Shearer, R.D., M.S., meet with us. Working together, my patient, the patient's family, Luz, and I construct a perfect dietary prescription based on patient needs and preferences. Only rarely do two patients receive the same diet. I will present the information in this book so that you will be able to create a unique healing experience for yourself.

What I learned at the conference in Wyoming brought my knowledge and ability to help heal to a higher level. I learned the latest information on preventing and healing illness at the cellular level by using food to maintain genetic integrity. If you have been following the news about the human genome project, you are probably aware of the great advances it promises. One day, drugs or therapies will fight illness by treating our genes. But I believe we can do that right now by using food as our form of genetic therapy. My program will act on your body, your brain, your mind, and your spirit. It will also touch you on your deepest inner level: your soul. After all, mind, body, and spirit are united; they are one. True healing requires we affect them all. This is the future of medicine—and here we are together at this precious moment.

SPIRITUAL NUTRITION

Perhaps you are one of the many people today who are aware of the deep spiritual awakening occurring on the planet. You can see it in the latest best-selling books and seminars. Some of the most popular speakers of our day, such as my colleagues Dr. Deepak Chopra and Debbie Ford, bring a spiritual slant to everything they say and do. Take a look at Oprah Winfrey's show, the most popular program on daytime television, which has showcased many influential new authors and spokespersons for the benefits of a spiritual lifestyle. Each *Oprah* program ends with a segment called "Touching Spirit," which is very popular and empowering to the members of her audience. It stirs them at a deep level.

This kind of elevation in consciousness recently touched one of my healing partners, a forty-year-old woman named Jane, who had spent a lot of time searching for help in dealing with her serious case of chronic fatigue syndrome. Jane had visited some of the most highly regarded physicians in America but had made little progress. One renowned doctor saw her for fifteen minutes, glanced at her chart in a cursory way, and told her that he wasn't optimistic about her recovery. Despite that unpleasant experience, she kept searching for a cure—or at least someone who believed in her ability to heal. Finally, she was referred to me. Working together, Jane and I designed a program that returned her to wellness.

One day she wanted to discuss a realization she had had, based on her meditation practice and reinforced by her travels around the country. She felt that something important was happening in the minds of people, but she couldn't put her finger on it. She asked me if I knew what it was. I told her that I saw the situation as more than just a change from the old way of treating people medically to a new way. The real shift we are witnessing today, I said, and still believe, is in how we look at the world in relation to ourselves.

I have written about the reasons behind this shift before. As I discussed in my book *Meditation as Medicine,* we are now entering a new age: the Age of Aquarius. Age shifts are natural phenomena that occur every two thousand years. Jesus Christ ushered in the previous transition, from the Age of Sagittarius to the Age of Pisces. Astrological scholars believe that the world changed again at midnight on November 11, 1991. At that moment the Age of Pisces ended and the Age of Aquarius began. Astrological transitions are marked by three seven-year periods totaling a twenty-one-year cusp. This current transition will end in 2012. Each seven-year stage brings with it accelerated change. I think you will agree that we are certainly seeing such a positive change now as people become more aware of their spiritual nature. But we are also witnessing the polar opposite of that positive change. The negative corollary in this age of transition includes an increase in terrorism, fear, violence, and rage. On a medical level, we can see a rising incidence of illnesses such as chronic fatigue and obesity, as well as escalating rates of some cancers.

The single most significant change we are witnessing in this Age of Aquarius is how it revolves around experience rather than information. In its initial stages, the Age of Aquarius still centered on information and its effects on us. For example, our collective quest for information led to the development of the personal computer and the rise of the Internet. During the information age, the cry was "I want to know, I want to know." While it is still useful, the desire for pure information for its own sake has subsided as we realize that what we need most is useful personal experience. As we ride the crest of the second seven years of this cusp, a new impulse has emerged. Now the shout is "I want an experience." This is readily apparent in many aspects of modern life—in reality TV, for example, and in the increase in adventure travel.

This change in paradigm is especially vivid in the practice of medicine. Because patients have become so utterly discouraged with medical practice as driven by big business and HMOs, they now visit the offices of alternative medical practitioners in droves. In the 1980s, very few Americans had consulted an alternative medical practitioner, be it a nutritionist, yoga therapist, meditation expert, chiropractic physician, massage therapist, acupuncturist, or herbalist. However, in a 1991 Harvard study, this number had increased to 34 percent, and in 1999 over 50 percent of Americans had visited an alternative medical practitioner. This number is further climbing with every passing day. Extrapolation of the 1991 Harvard study suggests that Americans made an estimated 425 million visits to providers of alternative medicine in 1990 alone. The financial ramification of this shift to integrative medicine is staggering. Expenditures associated with unconventional medical therapy in 1990 were approximately $13.7 billion, three quarters of which was paid by patients out of their own pockets. These uninsured costs are now up to $27 billion, based on a survey reported recently by the *New England Journal of Medicine*.

The reason people are embracing integrative medicine is apparent. Patients crave the experience of wellness that this type of treatment gives. It is what I call the feeling of healing. You usually leave the office of an alternative medical doctor feeling a lot better than when you entered. You have hope and the experience of happiness. The practitioner usually spends quality time with you, asking questions and seeking feedback. It has been my experience that when conventional doctors see you they are rarely in the moment. Their minds seem to be elsewhere. Many people tell me that a trip to the doctor leaves them feeling like a number or a file, not a person. It's no wonder, then, that so many patients, even those with chronic illnesses, are bailing out of the system. For the most part, conventional medicine does little to provide them with a true healing experience.

However, because patients demand it, conventional medicine has been forced to integrate proven natural healing techniques into the standard care of surgery, radiation therapy, and drugs. Yet, there is still a long way to go. One reason the evolution toward alternative or holistic medicine becomes bogged down is that we are taught to rely on technology instead of on our lifestyles and ourselves to heal. We have been taught that optimal health, deep healing, satisfaction, gratification, happiness, and even God can be found out there somewhere. This concept of looking outside is simply not correct. All answers lie within. As long as words have been written, saints, sages, poets, writers, philosophers, and yogis have commented on this concept and shared this truth. About five hundred years ago, an Indian guru named Arjun clarified my favorite interpretation of this reality. He was known as the Fifth Master, the king of this world and the next. Here is what he wrote:

> All things are within the heart,
> The home of the self.
> Outside there is nothing.
> Those who look outside themselves
> Are left wandering in doubt.

Guru Arjun tells us that the truth we seek is within ourselves, and I agree. The answers to many of our greatest desires, needs, and longings are inside. We only need to learn how to retrieve them.

The most powerful vehicle for retrieving our longed-for answers is applied intelligence, which is the combination of information and experience. Applied intelligence brings true wisdom because it includes experience, usually on a deep level. Because times are changing, medicine must embrace change. It will do so for one simple reason: we, the people, want it to.

FORWARD TO THE FUTURE

In his best-selling book *Eating Well for Optimal Health,* Andrew Weil, M.D., outlined his seven basic principles of diet and health. I'd like to repeat them here for you:

- We have to eat to live.
- Eating is a major source of pleasure.
- Food that is healthy and food that gives pleasure are not mutually exclusive.
- Eating is an important focus of social interaction.
- How we eat reflects and defines our personal and cultural identity.
- How we eat is one determinant of health.
- Changing how we eat is one strategy for managing disease and restoring health.

From *Eating Well for Optimal Health* by Andrew Weil, M.D. Copyright 2000 by Andrew Weil, M.D. Used by permission of Alfred A. Knopf, a division of Random House, Inc.

I'm sure you will agree that all seven principles are reasonable and true. Nevertheless, I believe we can continue to go forward in our approach to food based on available new knowledge. We can begin with Dr. Weil's last principle and move beyond it with a new intensity. In the pages of this book, I will show you why it is so vitally important to leave your old nutritional habits of the past century behind and chart a new and different course. For example:

- I will tell you how food acts as a messenger to your genes and how you can use that knowledge to create vibrant health and healing.
- I will give you an introductory course on the latest scientific knowledge about why food is actually medicine for your body, mind, and spirit.
- I will share with you my new seven principles of eating a modern healing diet. You will learn about organic foods and determine how to identify them and where to find them. I will also tell you about the risks of genetically modified foods and how to avoid them.
- I will teach you how to gently and safely detoxify your body from the environmental pollutants you absorb every day.
- I will lead you to discover uncommon uses for common natural foods.
- I will teach you to craft special food combination diets for specific illnesses.
- I will teach you to use organic juices as natural medicines.
- I will show you how to institute specific vitamin and herbal therapies to accelerate healing.
- I will provide you with innovative recipes for meals that heal. Many of them come from my own family. My wife, Kirti, is Italian, and she is a wonderful cook. My son, Sat, is a professional natural food chef. My daughter, Hari, is a graduate of the New Mexico School of Natural Therapeutics. All of them have happily agreed to share some of their cooking ideas. Finally, with the blessings of my teacher, Yogi Bhajan, and his talented wife, Bibiji, I will instruct you on the preparation of spiritual nutrition recipes from the ancient healing tradition of yoga nutritional therapy.

You will be asked to complete various assignments during the course of the book to determine your intake of food and help design the best diet for your ailment, issue, or concern. The first interactive exercise will begin at the end of this chapter. At various times I will also suggest that you log onto my website, www.drdharma.com, to explore further information, such as a complete list of non–genetically engineered foods, which space limitations prohibit me from listing fully in the text of this book.

YOGA NUTRITIONAL THERAPY

Yoga nutritional therapy originated in India over five thousand years ago and was brought to the West in 1969 by Yogi Bhajan. He taught these time-tested nutritional techniques along with the ancient (and formerly secret) sacred science of kundalini yoga and meditation.

Yoga nutritional therapy differs from Ayurvedic medicine in that the former doesn't require you to understand the three different body types: kapha, pitta, and vata. Unless you take the time to really study Ayurveda or go to an experienced qualified practitioner, which can be very difficult to find, you may not be able to fully benefit from the Ayurvedic method. But healing doesn't have to be so complicated. Everything you need for self-restoration can be found in this book. Understanding and using yoga nutritional therapy is actually very easy.

In yoga nutritional therapy, there is little distinction between food as basic nutrition and food as medicine. This system intertwines highly developed aspects of healing and cuisine. It is a true delight for my wife and me to dine with Yogi Bhajan and Bibiji. Bibiji is an outstanding food-as-medicine cook as well as the author of two cookbooks. Thanks mostly to her, meals at their home are memorably tasty, optimally healing, and easy to digest. At a time when so many people are seeking a return to a more natural way of living, nutritional healing is becoming more popular. Hence the saying by Yogi Bhajan, "Doctors diagnose, food cures, and God heals." If you follow the advice I give in this book, you can reap the benefits of nutritional healing for yourself.

FOOD LOG EXERCISE #1

To start on your way, keep a food log for three days. You will be delighted by the information you'll gain about yourself. It is the perfect way to begin your healing journey.

In addition to noting the foods you eat, pay attention to how you feel shortly after you eat. Answer these questions:

1. Do you feel awake, with enhanced energy?
2. Do you feel tired after eating?
3. Do you have any bloating in your stomach, or gas?
4. Any pain or stiffness in your joints?
5. How is your sleep? Is it better, worse, or the same?
6. Does eating give you brain fog, or do you feel sharp and alert?
7. How does what you eat affect your libido?

Here is a sample food log for you to use:

Date: _____

Breakfast: _____

How I felt: _____

Snack (if any): _____

Lunch: _____

How I felt: _____

Snack: _____

Dinner: _____

End with a summary of the day's eating experience.

CHAPTER 2

What Signals Are You Sending
to Your Body?

I never knew my father. He and my mother divorced when I was a baby. Later he remarried and had a son, my half brother, David. He and I met only once before, and now here we are getting together in a San Francisco hotel after a hiatus of close to twenty years. I sit opposite him in awe because in many ways I feel as though I'm looking in a mirror. Well, not exactly, because he's much taller than I am and has dark hair, while I'm fair. But it's spooky because he makes the same hand gestures I make, so it's as if I'm looking at a mirror image. Not only that, his hands could be mine— they're the same shape. And that mouth—it's my smile. I also discover that I have been wrong all these years about where I got my sensitivity. For some reason I always believed that it came from my mother. After spending some time with David, I'm convinced that it's at least partly from my father as well. I'm getting a firsthand lesson on the power of our genes.

If you're like most people, you believe that your genes have predetermined just about everything about you. As you look in the mirror each morning perhaps you see your mother's eyes or your father's smile. You may also be convinced that your genes have already predetermined the illnesses you are destined to suffer. In her book *Living Downstream*, Dr. Sandra Steingraber described her health challenges in living with bladder cancer. Because her mother, uncle, and grandfather had all died of various forms of cancer, many people who knew Sandra assumed that she had inherited cancer genes. They weren't aware that Sandra had been adopted. Her cancer, she believed, was caused by exposure to environmental pollution as a

12

child. This reminds us of the fundamental truth where supposed genetic predispositions are concerned: external conditions—the circumstances to which your genes are exposed—contribute either to maximum wellness or to disease, accelerated aging, and premature death.

I live and work in Tucson. Not long ago I opened our daily paper, *The Citizen,* and read the story of Vernon White, who served in Vietnam in the late 1960s. Along with tens of thousands of other soldiers, Vern was doused with Agent Orange, the infamous and highly toxic herbicide used to clear ground cover in the dense jungles. According to the Department of Defense, as many as 19 million gallons of Agent Orange were dumped on Vietnam. Our government admits that the toxin is responsible for the terminal lung cancer from which Vern suffers. His exposure to Agent Orange injured his genes beyond their ability to repair themselves, and cancer was the result. Agent Orange has been proved to be the cause of at least ten other types of fatal cancers in the same way—by ruining good genes.

If you think that we're programmed in advance by our genes to have cancer or not, the sad story of Vernon White shows that this isn't always the case. He had excellent genes until Agent Orange came along. The Stockholm Study augments this knowledge. In that research study, over one thousand identical twins were observed for many years. At the end of that time it was noted that there was no correlation between the illnesses the twins developed. One of a pair might have developed heart disease, the other cancer.

Many people aren't aware of this type of work, however. A recent survey conducted by the American Institute for Cancer Research highlights this point. Eighty-six percent of people in the survey thought that genes cause cancer. According to leading researchers, however, only about 10 to 15 percent of cancers are genetic in origin; the rest are caused by a combination of environmental and lifestyle factors.

HOW FOOD AFFECTS YOUR GENES

The food you eat is among the most significant factors affecting your genes and pushing them toward cancer by causing mutation or disruption in their function. That is, what you eat can either prevent cancer and other chronic illnesses or help cause them.

Consider the following: Imagine that you are sitting in a lecture hall where I am at the podium discussing food as medicine. During the course of the lecture I announce that I have a guest outside the room. I describe him as a fifty-five-year-old man who works twelve hours a day, eats junk food, smokes two packs of cigarettes a day, drinks alcohol to excess, doesn't exercise, practices no stress management techniques, and has no social support system or genuine faith. Do you anticipate seeing someone who looks younger or older than his chronological years? You'd guess that he would look older, and you'd almost certainly be right.

Before he comes out, I announce the presence of another fifty-five-year-old. This one is happy with his life. He wakes up every morning and, as he says, "I shake hands with God." He eats well, following a primarily vegetarian diet with some fish; he loves organic produce, doesn't smoke or drink, and plays tennis four times a week, after which he lifts weights. He is very content with his family and has a strong and genuine spiritual life. How old do you imagine he'd look? Younger than his years, correct?

Finally, both men come out of hiding, and both your guesses prove to be right. The first man looks seventy, and the second looks forty-five. There is a quarter of a century difference between them, judging by looks alone. The first man has done everything he could to push his genes to express themselves in a negative way, while the second has encouraged his genes toward the expression of optimal well-being. They have had a choice—a say in what their genes would and would not do. The same choice now faces you.

Because you eat so often, your food is the single most important way to maintain your genetic integrity or to destroy it. Many excellent scientific studies underscore this vitally important truth. Richard Weindruch, Ph.D., has conducted research into how genes are affected by dietary change. The results were published in *Scientific American* in 1996. His paper, "Nutrient Modulation of Gene Expression," illustrates that simply by reducing the number of total calories eaten, the life span of a lab mouse could be prolonged by 30 percent. In human terms, that would translate into extending the predicted life span from an average of seventy-six years to a ripe old ninety-three. You'd be very satisfied with that life expectancy, wouldn't you? I'd gladly settle in advance for ninety-some good years.

There are 6,347 genes in the typical lab rat. Dr. Weindruch discovered that during normal aging, when the animal was permitted to eat as much as it desired, 5 percent of the rat's genes underwent an increase in activity and

5 percent decreased. Ninety percent of the rat's genes showed no change in activity levels. Are you surprised to learn that the 5 percent that rose in activity were stress genes, and the 5 percent that fell were energy genes? This is similar to what I see in patients who are aging prematurely. They are fatigued, depressed, and stressed. They describe having chronic pain, arthritis, memory loss, and weak immune systems. Some are recovering from cancer. Unfortunately, until I ask, they have rarely thought about how diet may have caused many of their symptoms.

The rats in Dr. Weindruch's study that ate all they wanted experienced more stress and less energy. The opposite was true among the rats that ate less. They maintained their youthful biochemistry even as they aged. Their fur was shiny, they were sexually active, and they did not have arthritis, cancer, or memory loss.

Perhaps you aren't interested in being able to run a maze at age sixty, but I know you would like to have as much energy as possible, and you want to be active at every age and stage of life. Merely by cutting down on your total calories and eating better foods, you can send positive signals to your genes, thereby increasing your chances for a long, robust life.

Other researchers, most notably Roy Walford, M.D., a retired professor of pathology at UCLA, have conducted similar research on larger animals, such as monkeys, and even humans. The results were similar. Walford's research showed that theoretically a person can live for approximately 120 years without a severe decline in quality of life. His research in the famous Biosphere I experiment, which took place about fifty miles from my desert home, also showed that eating a low-calorie diet decreased the activity of cholesterol genes and thus reduced fats in the blood that are associated with heart disease.

As a doctor, specializing in brain longevity, I can tell you that Dr. Walford's research also has very important implications for cognitive function. Eating well modulates the genes that regulate the production, as well as the quality and quantity, of the important brain chemicals known as neurotransmitters, such as serotonin and dopamine. As a result, you can eat to prevent or reverse memory loss and influence mood. Using food as an anti-aging medicine helps your brain to keep regenerating for as long as you live. I have seen this many times in my clinical practice.

Dr. Walford and his life extension enthusiasts eat approximately 1,500 to 2,000 calories a day. This is less than most men are used to eating—but then, again, in the United States we eat too much. This is quite obvious to me when I travel to Europe or Asia, where the portions at mealtime are much smaller than those we serve here, and as a result the level of obesity is low. I recently saw a picture of Dr. Walford, and at seventy-five he looks at least twenty years younger. He's very active physically, jogging every day. Intellectually, too, he's active, busily writing and speaking in public about his work.

The key to the Walford plan is what he calls undernutrition without malnutrition. This means being able to comfortably lower your caloric intake without sacrificing nutrient density or the positive messages that your food sends to your genes. In this book, almost all the recipes for food as medicine follow that concept. They are first and foremost nutrient dense, and many of them are low in calories as well.

All the research on caloric restriction points out that you are constantly speaking to your genes, and the words are the food you eat. On the surface of all your cells there are receptors, or chemical and vibrational handles. These receptors are attuned to the energetic intelligence pervading their environment—your body. Moment to moment, your body is buzzing with signals of peace or stress. These signals can be vibrational, chemical, nutritional, or hormonal. Regardless of the form they take, they are transmitted as part of the vast intelligence network linking mind, body, and spirit.

After a message is picked up by a cell's receptors, the machinery inside the cell responds by synthesizing certain chemicals called second messengers. These messengers then communicate with the nucleus in the center of the cell, where the genes are housed. These genes pick up the signal, and, based on the message received—peace or stress—they synthesize proteins, such as enzymes, and other chemicals, such as cytokines and leukotrienes, that are then sent out of the cell as messenger molecules. These new chemical messengers communicate with other cells all over your body. This is the basis of the science of intercellular communication, the optimal functioning of which is crucial to total health and longevity.

HEALTHY FOODS, UNHEALTHY FOODS, AND YOUR BODY

The various components of food, which we will cover later in this book, send messages of health or illness to your genes. And whether you can hear it or not, your genes talk back. The subtle sounds coming deep from within your 30 trillion dancing cells echo something like this: "I really like what's happening here. This is cool. I'm going to continue to produce good molecules and make this a bliss experience." Or, if you're eating food that troubles your genes, the inner message may indicate a dysfunction, something like this: "Hey, what's going on here? I have many ways of expressing my potential, and now I'm so stressed I need to express it with hostility. I'm under siege. I'm being fed a pile of junk, and I don't really like that. So, I'm going to put this body into an alarm state. Push the stress buttons! Pump out the adrenaline and cortisol! Get to those battle stations!"

The second situation, that of chronic high-level arousal, is the one many of my patients have been experiencing for years. Chronic stress produces millions of free radicals, those damaging by-products of metabolism. Free radicals injure DNA, causing gene mutations that lead to cancer. The negative signal received by DNA from free radicals may also cause the production of other chemicals such as prostaglandins, which create the inflammation that leads to arthritis and many other illnesses, including Alzheimer's (see chart below). Finally, this negative cascade of unhealthy food leading to cellular injury may also affect your lipid chemistry, which can lead to heart disease, also an illness of inflammation.

SERIOUS DISEASES RELATED TO CHRONIC INFLAMMATION

Cancer: Chronic inflammation is a finding in most cancers.

Heart attack: Chronic inflammation leads to coronary disease.

Alzheimer's: Chronic inflammation kills brain cells.

Stroke: Chronic inflammation promotes blood clots.

Arthritis: Inflammatory cytokines destroy joint cartilage.

Kidney failure: Inflammatory molecules damage kidney cells.

Asthma: Inflammation closes airways.

Allergy: Inflammation induces autoimmune reaction.

Pancreatitis: Inflammation injures pancreas cells.

Fibrosis: Inflammatory cytokines attack traumatized tissue.

Surgical complications: Inflammatory cytokines prevent healing.

Anemia: Blood cell production is hindered by inflammation.

Fibromyalgia: Inflammation, inflammation, inflammation.

Other intercellular messengers released as a result of faulty nutrition include the stress hormone cortisol; the sex hormones estrogen, testosterone, and DHEA; and insulin, the hormone of blood sugar control. Research has shown that these intercellular communicators can keep your body in healthy balance or lead to disease, depending on how your genes respond to the nutrition they receive from the food you eat.

Signs That Your Cells May Be Receiving Damaging Communication from Unhealthy Foods

Symptom	Cellular Miscommunication
Obesity	Improper fat storage message
Glucose intolerance	Insulin imbalance
Depression	Neurotransmitter dysfunction
Inflammation of joints, muscles, or organs	Increased genetic production of inflammatory proteins
Attention deficit disorder (ADD)	Impaired neurotransmitters
Elevated LDL ("bad") Cholesterol	Imbalanced fat metabolism
Excessive free radicals	Increased injurious chemicals
Frequent colds, possible cancer	Impaired immune chemicals
Headache	Increase in various chemical mediators
Chronic fatigue	Poorly regulated energy
Fibromyalgia	Impaired pain signals

From *Improving Intracellular Communication in Managing Chronic Illness* by Jeffrey S. Bland. Excerpted with permission of the Institute for Functional Medicine, 5800 Southview Drive, Gig Harbor, WA 98335, the copyright holder.

In his book *Journey Into Healing,* Deepak Chopra writes:

> The body is not a frozen sculpture.
> It is a river of information—
> A flowing organism empowered
> By millions of years of intelligence.
> Every second of our existence
> We are creating a new body.

How you eat now tells your genes what type of body you want to have later.

Back at the turn of the 20th century, disease was deep down, dark, and slow. Because antibiotics had yet to be invented, illnesses such as pneumonia and tuberculosis were common. In fact, my maternal grandfather died of pneumonia at the age of forty-three in 1922.

Disease today is characterized by speed, just as our society is. We have unregulated cell growth, which we call cancer, and overgrowth, which we call obesity. In many cases, there is a proven relationship between the two. For example, some risk factors for colon cancer are obesity, excessive consumption of red meat, and lack of exercise.

I believe very strongly that there is a connection between our fast-paced, nanosecond-oriented world and the prevalent diseases of today. Simply put, life moves at a much greater pace than ever before, and most people have not yet evolved to the point where their nervous systems are strong enough to handle it. Your neurons have to deal with far more information and arousal than ever before. This might not be quite so challenging if you had Albert Einstein's brain or a supercomputer on your shoulders, but essentially you have the same gray matter your ancestors had ten thousand or more years ago.

We now have instant news, instant money, instant war, instant communication, instant information, and instant gratification. We manage many chores at the same time, calling it multitasking. We have land phones, cell phones, pagers, electronic mail, snail mail, and hand-held computers. All these technological gadgets have been invented to help us be more productive.

But becoming so productive has given us a new deficiency disease— one not curable with a vitamin, nutrient, or food. We are suffering from a severe deficiency of free time. Most working Americans are allowed only a few weeks of vacation each year. This does not compare to vacations in other countries, principally in Europe, where workers are encouraged to enjoy six weeks of annual vacation. Moreover, sleep deprivation is a major medical problem. In my practice, a patient who sleeps well is rare indeed.

Because of our deficiency of free time, using food as peaceful medicine is of paramount importance to bring balance back to your life. If you constantly push your body's limits nutritionally, you speed up the aging of your body, mind, and spirit. High-frequency stress foods are those that cause an alarm reaction in the body. I'm talking about white sugar, refined foods without fiber, red meat, caffeine, alcohol, and others I list below. They all cause a signal of artificial stimulation to be relayed to your genes. Your genes receive the hurry-up signal—and they obey. Unfortunately, what is really being hurried along is the development of illness and perhaps even death.

ALARM FOODS

White foods (sugar, white bread, flour, cake, pasta, milk, white rice)

Alcohol

Artificial sweeteners

Cheese

Red meat

Processed foods

Bacon

Salami

Lunch meats

Pork

Hot dogs

Fast food

Soft drinks

Caffeine

Butter

Margarine

Coconut oil, palm oil

Safflower, sunflower, cooked sesame, corn, soy, and cottonseed oils

Unskinned, non–free-range poultry

Non–free-range eggs

These alarm foods all have in common a high fat content, the majority of which is of the saturated variety. Saturated fats, such as those found in red meat, are associated with increased risk of diseases such as heart disease, cancer and Alzheimer's. Clearly, the kind of fat you eat has a major influence on your health and longevity. Foods containing omega-3 (the "good" fat), such as salmon, tuna, olive oil, and flaxseed oil, inhibit inflammation. Foods high in saturated fats stimulate the formation of inflammation molecules. They are also unusually high in nutrient-weak calories, whereas nutrient-dense calories are what we need to ensure ourselves a healthy life expectancy.

What signals are you sending to your body? Do you eat alarm foods that create a buzz of false energy so you can survive your fast-paced life? If so, the legacy you are creating may include disease because of how your genes will respond. The good news is that you, with your diet, can reverse the course of premature aging and the development of disease. You speak to your genes many times every day through the food you eat. Why not send them a healing signal?

FOOD LOG EXERCISE #2

1. What similarities do all alarm foods have?
2. After reading the list of alarm foods, notice which ones you eat most often.
2. Try to eliminate from your diet as many white alarm foods as you can.
3. Notice how you start to feel.

CHAPTER 3

Phytonutrients: How Vegetables and Fruits Act as Medicine

There is no reason why you can't live to your optimal potential as a perfect individual created in the image of God. How you relate to food and how you use it in your life can help you become that healthy, happy, complete human being.

Food is the original and best medicine. Today, this idea has become one of the guiding principles of healthy living. Every schoolchild has been taught that an apple a day keeps the doctor away, and I don't know anyone who would argue with the wisdom of that phrase. Apples are very healthy. They are rich in fiber, which promotes optimal gastrointestinal health. Apples also contain high amounts of natural vitamins and minerals, as well as the nutrient pectin, which contains soluble fiber and has been shown to fight high cholesterol levels and colon cancer. In fact, recent published reports reveal that improvements in diet and lifestyle may reduce the incidence of colon cancer by a whopping 70 percent.

Incorporating the concept of food as medicine into your life is a very practical decision because of the way specific foods activate your body's natural healing force. When this takes place—when you eat certain foods in a carefully chosen way—you are able to prevent and heal scores of ailments safely and effectively.

TECHNOLOGICAL MEDICAL ADVANCES ONLY GO SO FAR

A sixty-five-year-old politician has a severe heart attack. As part of a research protocol, he is offered a new type of medical procedure that his doctor thinks may save his life. The patient assumes that it involves surgery and tells the doctor, in a joking manner, to just put a zipper in his chest. "You never know," the man says. "The way things are going, you might have to go back in again."

The doctor tells him that yes, the procedure involves some surgery, but not that type. "We are going to make a small incision down to your spinal cord and withdraw some cells," the doctor explains. "They are stem cells, which can grow into any type of organ. We will then prepare them in a way that will allow us to inject them into your heart. Our theory is that this will allow your heart to grow new cells and reverse the effects of your heart attack." The patient agrees to the procedure. The operation is a success, but the man soon dies.

Even after the massive coronary attack and the surgical procedure, the politician kept on with the same hard-driving lifestyle as before. Most importantly, he did not change his high-fat, high-sugar, alarm-foods diet. Instead, he continued down the path of self-destruction, armed only with his knife and fork.

I don't believe that the future of medicine is in technology. Neither are the greatest discoveries of modern medical research to be found in the billion-dollar drugs that are pushed at us by multinational pharmaceutical giants, who seduce us with TV commercials. Nor does the future of health belong to the race to teach stem cells to regenerate new brain, pancreas, liver, or heart cells.

Rather, the future of good health will be found in the same place it has always existed: in the distinct chemical constituents of fruits and vegetables. When consumed on a regular basis, these "drugs" can do more than any magic bullet medicine, vaccine, or genetic twist to prevent and help treat heart disease, cancer, diabetes, Alzheimer's disease, arthritis, and the other scourges of our time.

That may sound like an outrageous statement if you are unfamiliar with the new medical discoveries I am about to describe or the practical advice that will follow. But, as I will show, it's all true.

GETTING BACK TO THE SOURCE

Everywhere I look I see the hand of God, especially in the natural bounty that grows on the earth. The One Creator—the same energy that causes a bird to migrate to the south in the winter, sets the sun to rise in the east every morning, and causes the stars to shine at night—has made it a priority to insure your divine well-being. Everything you need to help you fulfill your birthright of being healthy, happy, and whole is here for you, but you have strayed so far from the garden that you may no longer be able to see it. Moreover, our modern lifestyle focuses on technology, not Mother Nature. I hope that by spending the time and energy to travel down this road with me, you will enjoy your reward of glowing maximum health, utmost happiness, and a peaceful spirit.

So, let us begin—with vegetables. The vegetable kingdom provides many of the chemical nutrients your body needs to sustain and regenerate itself. You have a veritable pharmacy in your kitchen.

Vegetables and fruits prevent your genes from sending negative messages to the rest of the body. That is their most powerful and important medical effect. Beyond that, a diet rich in fruits and vegetables will lower your intake of fat, cholesterol, and refined sugar. You will increase your consumption of the all-important disease-fighting antioxidants and anti-inflammatory protective compounds, which are the keys to preventing cancer, heart disease, and chronic pain. Remember that the diet of fast food and processed food that so many Americans follow is a relatively recent phenomenon—about fifty years old at most. Our genes are suited to a diet of freshness, the way nature intended for us to eat. It's no wonder, then, that there is a disconnect between what some of us eat and what our cells expect to be fed. This disconnect, in great measure, is the cause of all disease.

THE NATIONAL INSTITUTES OF HEALTH AND "FIVE A DAY"

In September of 1999, the National Institutes of Health (NIH) published a "five a day" report, which advised all Americans to eat at least five servings of fruit and vegetables each and every day. According to the NIH, there was ample evidence that following this prescription would protect our health. At a total cost to taxpayers of over $40 million, the NIH instituted a mass media educational campaign. It wasn't hugely successful in changing our behavior—only 3.7 percent more Americans ate five daily servings of fruits and vegetables as a result—but the campaign did raise public awareness of the importance of fresh fruits and vegetables. The "five a day" mantra set the stage for further research in this area by other organizations, such as the American Institute for Cancer Research (AICR).

The AICR has done an outstanding job of satisfying its mission by emphasizing the importance of fresh foods in cancer prevention. Every year the group holds at least one major conference in Washington, D.C., to share the results of the latest research in this field. The AICR also sponsors other conferences around the country for cancer survivors as well as for the general public. Most important, however, is its strong commitment to funding innovative nutritional research at major medical institutions. The group has also published *Food, Nutrition and the Prevention of Cancer: A Global Perspective.* This book, co-sponsored by the *World Cancer Research Foundation,* has helped change the face of cancer research. While the lion's share of total research money still goes to the development of new drugs and technologies, the fact that nutritional research is now being funded to such a degree represents a breakthrough.

More useful knowledge will come from the nutritional research being underwritten by organizations like the AICR than will ever come from the development of poisons to kill cancer cells. With these drugs, the cure is sometimes worse than the disease. Think about it: If the poisons are capable of killing cancer cells, which are the fastest-growing cells in the body, they must also be able to kill a lot of other very useful cells along the way. This includes gastrointestinal cells, immune cells, and, obviously, hair follicles. Patients receiving chemotherapy are poisoned. Many can't even eat because of the nausea, and they may be prone to infections, fatigue, and weakness as a result of treatment. Does this sound like the road to health?

But the greatest thing the AICR has done is to increase the five-a-day recommendation of the NIH to seven a day: seven daily servings of fruits and vegetables. You need to eat that quantity of fruits and vegetables to obtain sufficient amounts of the medical ingredients they provide. Food is medicine, and as with drugs there is a proper dose.

PHYTONUTRIENTS

The active components of fruits and vegetables are called phytonutrients. They are the chemical compounds in plants that act on human cells and genes to bolster your body's innate defenses against illness. Put simply, phytonutrients can save your life.

It was only in 1986 that laboratory researchers began discovering dozens of "new" chemicals in common fruits and vegetables. In test tubes and in animal studies, these obscure compounds showed a remarkable ability to stop cancer. Today, our knowledge of phytonutrients is exploding. And as more is learned, we can say with confidence that the future of healing is not in drugs, vaccines, or stem cells. It is in food. As cancer specialist Mitchell Gaynor, M.D., told *Newsweek,* eating the right foods is "as specific to stopping cancer before it starts as wearing a seat belt is to lowering your risk of a fatal automobile accident."

Because of environmental exposure to toxins such as air pollution, first-hand and secondhand cigarette smoke, and several cancer-promoting chemicals in food and water, as well as the damage being done to your body by all kinds of internal and external stress, your own natural defenses are becoming overwhelmed. They need all the help they can get from phytonutrients. While I do believe in taking supplements both as insurance and for therapeutic purposes, my number one recommendation to my consultation healing partners and to you, my reading healing partner, is to eat a rainbow of fresh fruits and vegetables every day.

I know none of us is perfect. It's hard to break old habits and adopt new ones, even when they hold such awesome promise. However, when I began to eat more fruits and vegetables, my health—which was good to begin with—improved tremendously. I have seen hundreds of patients make remarkable health recoveries and lose weight when they did the same.

FOOD LOG EXERCISE #3

For three days, keep a record of all the fruits and vegetables you eat. Are you getting your seven a day?

CHAPTER 4

Vegetables as Medicine

I could present the information in this chapter simply by advising you to consume plenty of the chemical compounds sulforaphane, isothiocyanates, allicin, and epigallocatechin gallate. In case you didn't realize it, I just listed the names of the medically active components in common produce, the plant-based foods that contain all the phytonutrients you need to ward off and even cure many ailments, from upset stomach to cancer. Instead, I've compiled a far more useful glossary of common vegetables and their benefits for you.

BROCCOLI

Broccoli is by far the subject of the most exciting scientific food story of our time. It is difficult to overestimate broccoli's healing power. This cruciferous vegetable has been proved effective as a food medicine against cancer, heart disease, and a host of other serious conditions.

For many years we have known of broccoli's power as a cancer preventive. Today we have fresh evidence that backs broccoli as a major cancer fighter as well. We even know the exact spot of the broccoli plant that is best to eat. Paul Talalay, M.D., Distinguished Service Professor of Pharmacology and Director of the Laboratory for Molecular Sciences at Johns Hopkins University School of Medicine, recently expanded our knowledge about one of the major phytonutrients broccoli contains: sulforaphane. Sulforaphane triggers natural cancer-blocking agents in the body.

Dr. Talalay's research has shown that sulforaphane protects genes from damage by helping rid your body of harmful stress and alarm signal molecules. In a study done by Dr. Talalay and a colleague, Thomas Kensler, Ph.D., Professor of Environmental Health Sciences in the School of Public Health at Johns Hopkins, 145 laboratory animals were exposed to a strong cancer-causing chemical. Rats fed an extract of broccoli-containing sulforaphane and then exposed to the strong carcinogen were far less likely to develop cancer than were rats on a standard diet. After 50 days, 68 percent of the unprotected animals had breast tumors, compared with only 26 percent of those given the protective sulforaphane. Furthermore, when the broccoli-eating rats did develop cancer, their tumors were smaller and took longer to grow than those in the other rats.

Broccoli is particularly helpful in preventing cancers of the colon, breast, and prostate, according to other researchers. Most recently, scientists at the American Health Foundation discovered that sulforaphane inhibited the formation of premalignant lesions in the colons of rats. Furthermore, researchers in Toulouse, France, found that sulforaphane actually caused human cancer cells to die.

Exactly how does broccoli help us prevent and fight off cancer? In your cells, you have what are called phase I and phase II detoxification enzyme systems, which must be kept in delicate balance. Phase I enzymes search for cancer-causing compounds that have entered the body (through diet or environment) and make them easier to eliminate by turning them into water-soluble compounds or rendering them inactive in some other way.

Occasionally, however, phase I enzymes generate chemicals that are themselves carcinogenic. Hence the need for phase II enzymes, such as gluthathione S-transferase, which help the body detoxify the carcinogens produced by phase I enzymes. Phase II enzymes can also attack the carcinogens directly, destroy them, and escort them from the body before they can inflict genetic damage in your cells.

Sulforaphane prevents cancer by activating both detoxifying enzyme systems and also by causing cancer cell death. According to Dr. Talalay, "We now have evidence that the anti-cancer potential of components in cruciferous vegetables like broccoli—and particularly in broccoli sprouts—is longer lasting, more potent, more versatile, and ultimately safer than we ever expected."

Why did Dr. Talalay recommend that we eat broccoli sprouts? His research team discovered that as the broccoli plant grows older, the concentration of sulforaphane decreases. Young plants, such as three-day-old sprouts, yield much greater cancer-fighting power. In fact, his research demonstrated that certain varieties of three-day-old broccoli sprouts contain 20 to 50 times the concentration of sulforaphane as the mature cooked vegetable. On average, it was found that one ounce of broccoli sprouts provide as much cancer-fighting activity as twenty ounces of mature, cooked broccoli—that's twenty times the concentration.

Recall that sulforaphane activates the phase II enzyme called glutathione S-transferase. Studies show that high levels of this enzyme in gastrointestinal tissue protect against a wide range of cancers. Sulforaphane was also shown to inhibit negative, chemically induced DNA changes by as much as 80 percent. Sulforaphane, therefore, may prevent lung cancer because of its effect in fighting environmentally induced cancers.

Broccoli also contains a little known but incredibly important detoxification enzyme called D-glucarate. Studies in animals indicate that it may be effective in inhibiting the formation of cancer and its progression. The preliminary results of human studies are equally impressive. Extrapolation of these data reveals that the D-glucarate found in broccoli may significantly lower your risk of cancers of the breast, bladder, lung, skin, colon, prostate, and liver.

How Sulforaphane Drives Cancer Agents Out of Human Cells

1 When a carcinogenic molecule from food, drink, air, or smoke invades a cell, its cancer-causing potential can kick in.

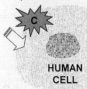

HUMAN CELL

Within minutes of being eaten, sulforaphane, a cancer-fighting phytochemical, enters the bloodstream and rapidly boosts the body's antioxidant defense systems.

Upon reaching a cell, the sulforaphane activates a group of proteins called Phase 2 enzymes.

3 The activated Phase 2 enzymes then "disarm" the carcinogenic molecule and thereby accelerate its removal from the cell.

2

Dr. Talalay is now at work on clinical trials that attempt to determine how broccoli sprout extracts and other plant foods can be cultivated, prepared, and consumed for optimum defense against cancer and other diseases. Imagine that: broccoli medicine! He has founded the Brassica Chemoprotection Laboratory within Johns Hopkins University to study this topic. The sprouts developed through his research at Hopkins are now available to the general public as BroccoSprouts. They're sold primarily in health food stores next to alfalfa sprouts, which they resemble.

In light of Dr. Talalay's findings, perhaps to our mothers' and grandmothers' advice to "Eat your vegetables" we should add "Eat your sprouts!"

BEETS

Beets get their color from beta-cyanin, a promising cancer fighter. They are also rich in folic acid, which is crucial for maximum cardiovascular and brain health, and potassium, which is important for muscle function and general metabolic activity.

According to yoga nutritional therapy, women can benefit from eating beets during their menstrual cycle because it replenishes the iron lost in the blood. For that reason, beets are also considered a useful adjunct in the treatment of iron-deficiency anemia. Beets are also a wonderful liver tonic.

Meanwhile, remember to buy beets with their greens attached. When you get home, cut off the stalks at ½ inch from the base and store them separately to help them stay fresher. The stalks are best consumed within 2 to 3 days in salads. When you prepare the beets, remember to cook and eat the green stalks as well as the beets because both are very nutritious.

Please note that beets sometimes turn your urine and stools red. Rarely, this may indicate an iron deficiency; usually it's just a sign that the vegetable's metabolites have passed through your body.

Another great way to reap the benefits of beets is through juicing. Simply take fresh organic beets, wash and scrub them well, and insert them into your favorite juicer. As beet juice is very strong, I recommend using two ounces in an eight-ounce glass of apple and carrot juice.

BRUSSELS SPROUTS

Brussels sprouts are not true sprouts but mature vegetables. Like all members of the cabbage family, Brussels sprouts contain a phytonutrient called indole-3-carbinol. They also contain allyl isothiocyanite, which gives them their distinctive odor. Indole-3-carbinol works by blocking the effects of extra estrogen, which may promote breast cancer. Moreover, indole-3-carbinol stimulates the phase II enzyme system that helps clear cancer-causing toxins from your body.

Brussels sprouts have been shown to reduce the risk of breast, prostate, and colon cancer; lower cholesterol and the risk of heart attack; and eliminate constipation. Women using birth control pills can also benefit from eating Brussels sprouts. Taking birth control pills may lead to folic acid deficiency, and Brussels sprouts contain a fair amount of immunity-boosting vitamin C and folic acid.

In a study done in the Netherlands in 1997, people who ate more than ten ounces of Brussels sprouts a day for three weeks displayed a 28 percent reduction in damage to their DNA, compared with those who ate none at all.

In a different study that shows the importance of eating fresh vegetables rather than canned ones, researchers came up with an ingenious plan. The challenge was to find a placebo similar to a Brussels sprout, because the subjects would surely know whether or not they were eating the vegetable. The scientists gave the study group a plate of lightly steamed, beautiful, fresh, organic Brussels sprouts, and the placebo group received formerly canned Brussels sprouts taken straight from the hospital cafeteria's steam table! Because the phytonutrients had been cooked and processed out of the canned Brussels sprouts, their nutritional value was close to zero, so they provided an excellent control group.

To obtain the best health benefits, buy your Brussels sprouts, and all other veggies, fresh. Also, try to pick Brussels sprouts that are the same size so they'll cook evenly. The leaves on the outside contain the most phytonutrients and should be left on unless they're damaged.

THE CABBAGE FAMILY, CAULIFLOWER, AND OTHER CRUCIFERS

Like all members of the crucifer family, cabbage and cauliflower are loaded with nutrients, especially indoles and sulforaphane. Savoy cabbage contains additional phytonutrients called beta-sitosterol, pheophytin-a, nonacosane, and nonacosanone, all of which are very potent cancer fighters. Bok choy, or Chinese cabbage, contains brassinin, another powerful estrogen-regulating nutrient that battles breast cancer.

Despite the great benefits of cauliflower, I do have a cautionary tale to share with you. One of my healing partners, a sixty-year-old banker, had suffered from gout for a decade. Recently, to lose weight and improve his overall health, he decided to eat more vegetables, especially cauliflower. After about a week he had an attack of gout in his feet. What he didn't realize is that cauliflower worsens gout because it contains amino acids called purines, which in the body become a compound called uric acid. The uric acid crystals lodged in the joints of his feet, causing pain and swelling.

I found a way to help him resolve this attack and totally eliminate his gout. I had him stop eating all red meat, which contains many more purines than cauliflower does. I also had him cut way back on cauliflower and suggested that he add other cruciferous vegetables such as broccoli sprouts, Brussels sprouts, and cabbage to his diet. He was able to maintain a high level of phytonutrients in his body and lose the gout entirely.

CARROTS

It is well known that carrots are extremely high in beta-carotene, which your body converts to vitamin A. Vitamin A helps the mucous membranes of your respiratory tract defend your lungs against bacterial and viral invasion. It also maintains an optimal detoxifying potential throughout the body.

What about the old wives' tale about the benefits of carrots for your eyes? That tale is correct. Carrots contain a broad mix of carotenoids, including lutein and zeaxanthin, which help prevent cataracts, macular degeneration, and night blindness. The first two ailments are seen primarily in older people, but night vision disturbances can begin in the early fifties. It may be possible to delay the development of night vision disturbances in later life by eating a wide variety of orange vegetables, especially carrots. These orange vegetables all contain vitamin A, and the more vitamin A you have in your body, the more rhodopsin you produce. Rhodopsin is a purple pigment that the eye needs in order to see in dim light.

The healthy properties of carrots are not the result of only the phytonutrients just named. Carrots contain additional antioxidants, including alpha-carotene, which fights cancer and heart disease. Carrots help prevent and treat heart disease because they are rich in calcium pectate, a soluble fiber that lowers cholesterol. Large population studies have shown that people with low levels of beta-carotene are more open to developing certain cancers, whereas those with higher levels of beta-carotene die of cancer much less often.

Eat your carrots with a little good fat, such as olive oil or a healthful ranch dressing, to aid in their absorption. If your new devotion to this vegetable turns your skin a faint shade of orange, don't worry—it's a harmless and transient condition called carotenosis. It is most common in children but also appears in adults. If this happens to you or your child, simply stop eating carrots for a few days and then begin enjoying them again, in moderation.

CHILI PEPPERS

Long before the rock group there was the vegetable: the original red-hot chili pepper. I must tell you that because I lived in New Mexico for over twenty years before moving full time to Arizona, I am totally prejudiced in favor of chili. Even now, whenever we go back to Albuquerque, Santa Fe, or Espanola, our first stop is at one of our favorite restaurants for a bowl of green chili.

Chilies raise your endorphin level. You feel so good after eating them that you want to eat more again—and soon. The reason God made chilies such bearers of good feelings is precisely that they are so good for you. They contain a tremendous amount of vitamin C and other antioxidant nutrients, including beta-carotene. Because they are so rich in vitamin C, chilies have been used as natural remedies for coughs, colds, sinusitis, and bronchitis around the globe. For centuries, healers from Mexico to India have known of these healing properties. There is even some evidence that chilies can help lower low-density lipoprotein (LDL), which we call bad cholesterol. As such, red or green chilies and jalapenos act as preventive medicine against strokes, high blood pressure, and heart attacks. They also help recovery from the common cold.

Before beginning my writing career I practiced anesthesiology and holistic pain management. I was founding director of the acupuncture, stress medicine, and chronic pain program at Maricopa Medical Center, the University of Arizona's teaching hospital in Phoenix. There, we used capsaicin, the phytonutrient in chili, to help treat chronic pain. It was prepared in a cream to be rubbed on the painful spot. People with arthritis found it was especially therapeutic when rubbed on aching joints. Capsaicin works by manipulating levels of substance P, a chemical that transmits pain sensations to the brain. The capsaicin depletes the nerve cells of this pain neurotransmitter. This cream, sold under various names in health food and drug stores, is very strong, so talk to your doctor or health care practitioner before using it, and be careful when applying it.

KALE

Kale is an outstanding source of many nutrients, including beta-carotene, calcium, iron, manganese, potassium, and vitamins C and E. Kale also contains high levels of the vision-protecting phytonutrient leutin. Although there are more than five hundred carotenoids, only fifty to sixty of them have been identified in food. The key carotenoids in kale are alpha-carotene, beta-carotene, gamma-carotene, beta-cryptoxanthin, leutin, lycopene, and zeaxanthin. These compounds neutralize free radicals and thereby help to protect the DNA in your genes. In the opinion of leading researchers and knowledgeable nutritionists, people who have lots of carotenoids in their diets tend to get less cancer.

PUMPKINS

Pumpkins are a terrific source of calcium, fiber, iron, and zinc, a key nutrient for prostate health and a strong immune system.

RED BELL PEPPERS

What a delightful surprise red bell peppers are. In addition to their great taste, red bell peppers contain three times the vitamin C of citrus fruit, such as oranges. They are also a great source of beta-carotene, fiber, and vitamin B_6. You may wonder why I prefer red bell peppers over green peppers. The answer is only time. When green peppers ripen on the vine, they turn red and their vitamin content increases. So bell peppers, just like some people and wines, get better with age. However, as they are on the top ten list of pesticide-laden vegetables when raised conventionally, I strongly suggest that you look for organic red bell peppers.

SPINACH

Spinach is among the best sources of folic acid, which is critically important for cardiovascular and brain health. Low folic acid levels in your blood are associated with high levels of the amino acid homocysteine. Excessive homocysteine is a marker for increased risk of death resulting from heart disease. And since heart disease is a strong risk factor for memory loss, high levels of homocysteine are a marker for Alzheimer's disease as well. A half cup of boiled spinach contains 131 micrograms of folic acid out of the 400 micrograms you need to eat every day to keep your homocysteine levels under control. Furthermore, in a recent report, neurologists recommended eating spinach three times a week as a brain tonic. As spinach is also on the top ten list of pesticide-laden vegetables when raised conventionally, I strongly suggest you look for organic spinach.

Spinach also contains a wide range of other nutrients, including beta-carotene, lutein, magnesium, manganese, the antioxidant quercetin, and vitamin K, which is essential for blood clotting. Spinach contains the perfect combination of minerals to help control the amount of water your body retains. It has a diuretic effect, which helps get rid of that bloated feeling that many of my patients say slows them down and keeps them from feeling truly fit. Spinach helps keep your blood pressure under control and also provides a healthy dose of iron to improve the blood.

Green leafy vegetables, including spinach, can supply adequate amounts of calcium and iron. And they don't come with any of the negatives associated with milk and red meat. Remember, milk and meat are both stimulating foods. They send alarm messages to your genes, which send stress signals throughout your body—and it is those signals of distress that accumulate over your lifetime and lead to illnesses such as heart disease and cancer.

SQUASH AND SWEET POTATOES

Squash and sweet potatoes, which are wonderful sources of fiber and vitamin E, also contain carotenoids, which are excellent antioxidants.

TOMATOES

One of my patients, an eighty-eight-year-old man, controls his prostate cancer by eating a whole can of cooked tomatoes every day. His urologist is amazed that his level of prostate-specific antigen (PSA), a marker of tumor size, has been falling thanks to this regimen. I believe it's because of lycopene, a very potent antioxidant found in tomatoes. Research into dietary lycopene suggests that it may lower the risk of heart attack and cancer. A study of more than 1,300 European men suggests that those consuming the most lycopene had half the risk of heart attack. A five-year study of 48,000 men found that those eating ten servings a week of cooked tomato products had the lowest risk of prostate cancer. Their risk was one third that of men eating fewer than two servings a week. Other studies suggest that lycopene may play a role in reducing the risk of other cancers, including cancers of the colon, rectum, and breast.

We aren't exactly sure how many servings of lycopene-rich foods you should eat each week. Some studies suggest seven to ten servings a week. A serving is equivalent to a half cup of tomato or spaghetti sauce, a quarter cup of tomato paste, or one medium tomato. Although usually high in fat, a slice of pizza is one serving as well. Whatever form of tomato you choose, it must be cooked to give you the maximum benefit.

TRINITY ROOT: GARLIC, ONIONS, AND GINGER

Ask any yoga nutritional therapist about the most important ingredients in the food-as-medicine lifestyle, and he or she will name the so-called trinity root. When Yogi Bhajan encapsulated his first herbal product over twenty years ago, he told his chief of staff, "Put garlic, onions, and ginger in the capsule. Otherwise no one will eat it." Trinity root is excellent for overall health maintenance or for help in recovering from illness—and it tastes good, too. A broth made of garlic, onions, and ginger root is a very good tonic, especially for fatigue. You can mix broccoli and Brussels sprouts with the trinity root, or just a few cloves of garlic, and steam them together to accelerate recovery from surgery. Trinity root is also considered by yogis to be a potency food for men and to increase sperm counts.

Although the use of trinity root for its myriad healing benefits goes back to the time of Pythagoras in ancient Greece, it has recently been the subject of research studies. The results show that the trinity root's reputation as a food with multiple healing properties is not unfounded.

Garlic, for example, which contains phytonutrients of the sulfur family, including diallyl disulfide, is useful as an antibacterial agent. It's also a potent force in reducing cholesterol and triglycerides. In fact, a review of sixteen studies involving 952 people showed that eating garlic, either fresh or powdered, decreased cholesterol by as much as 13 percent. By reducing cholesterol and triglycerides, you lower your risk of heart disease and stroke.

Garlic also contains a compound called S-allylcysteine, which scientists believe contains the vegetable's anticancer agent. A study of over 40,000 women living in the midwest revealed that those who ate garlic at least once a week had a 35 percent lower risk of colon cancer than those who didn't. Yogi Bhajan once suggested to a woman with breast cancer that she make a garlic pudding to augment her standard cancer therapy. She did, and she felt that it helped with her survival.

Onions are equally beneficial to your health. Because they contain quercetin, they are potent antioxidants. Onions also contain sulfur compounds, which lower cholesterol. So garlic and onions, when eaten regularly, either separately or together, are powerful fighters in the war on cancer and heart disease. Add to that some ginger root, the third member of trinity root, and it's almost a miracle food.

Ginger can help prevent motion sickness, soothe upset stomach, relieve migraines, ease arthritis pain because of its anti-inflammatory properties, and thin blood better than aspirin. I enjoy eating ginger at my favorite Japanese restaurant or having it in tea. Even ginger ale, which has very little actual ginger in it, is better than a regular soft drink to reduce stomach upset during a rough flight.

As the master, Yogi Bhajan, has said about the trinity root, "Onions, garlic, and ginger are not spices; they are the trinity roots of life. In yoga, people who do not take onions, garlic, and ginger are those who are not supposed to lead the life of a householder and are supposed to stay three miles away from where a woman dwells." In other words, for a man or a woman, eating the trinity root is necessary if you are to keep your feet on the ground while still living a spiritual life.

One of the best things about writing this book is that I have become inspired to eat all these multicolored vegetables. It's as though I am discovering the wonderment of good eating habits all over again.

Tonight I steamed a panoply of fresh vegetables in our rice cooker along with some Indian basmati rice. Then I put tomato sauce over it and added a tofu burger as a finishing touch. I used many of the veggies I've been discussing here: broccoli, carrots, Brussels sprouts, cauliflower, and red bell pepper. I enjoyed a delicious and healthy meal. I invite you to do the same. You can begin simply by trying Paola's carrot salad.

Paola's Carrot Salad
Makes 1 serving

1 medium carrot, grated
¼ finely chopped red bell pepper
1 tablespoon finely chopped green onion
2 teaspoons lemon juice
1 teaspoon extra virgin olive oil
pinch of sea salt or ½ teaspoon Braggs Liquid Aminos

Toss carrot, red pepper, and green onion with lemon juice, olive oil, and salt or Braggs. Serve with light, fresh cheese or cottage cheese and 1 slice of whole grain bread.

FOOD LOG EXERCISE #4

In your journal, take note of how you feel after eating the salad.

CHAPTER 5

Fruit as Medicine

I like to think of fruit and vegetables as yin and yang. For the most part, vegetables aren't sweet and are usually served later in the day. Fruit is sweet and light and is most often enjoyed in the morning. Because fruit contains comparable amounts of vitamins, minerals, fiber, and phytonutrients as vegetables, it is every bit as important in preventing cancer, heart disease, Alzheimer's, strokes, and arthritis. There is convincing scientific evidence that eating fresh fruit decreases cancer risk with no evidence to the contrary, according to the American Institute of Cancer Research.

APPLES

Apples contain a multitude of phytonutrients, including quercetin, which is found inside the apple and in its skin. Research has disclosed that men who eat one apple a day lower their risk of heart attack by 32 percent.

Pectin, the fiber in apples, helps keep your bowels regular and reduces the painful attacks of diverticulitis of the colon. There are more than 2,500 kinds of apples, and all are good for your health.

BANANAS

Bananas are high in potassium and therefore are useful if you get muscle cramps after exercise or with age. Also, patients who take diuretics for high blood pressure are usually advised by their doctors to eat a banana every day to replenish the potassium lost in urine. Bananas are also useful to treat ulcers; some scientists think they have an antibacterial effect that prevents ulcers from occurring. The smoothness of the fruit coats an upset stomach, too.

In yoga nutritional therapy, bananas are considered an excellent cleansing and rejuvenating food. I have suggested that patients eat up to ten a day in the spring to purify their systems. Bananas are also considered an essential ingredient of a woman's diet. Along with a bowl of steamed vegetables, a woman who wants to remain youthful for life should eat one banana every day (see Women's Health on p. 279). The phosphorus in the banana keeps a woman's metabolism functioning smoothly.

Remember to scrape the inside of the banana peel and either eat it directly or put it in a smoothie. The inner peel is rich in potassium, phosphorus, and antioxidants.

BERRIES

You may be surprised to learn that these little gems are powerful disease fighters. Name an illness, and one berry or another is effective at preventing it. Berries contain effective phytonutrients for the health of the eyes, brain, heart, and immune system. Berries are to fruit what broccoli is to vegetables. Is there any higher praise?

Berries contain quercetin, the powerful anticancer, anti-inflammatory, and cardioprotective antioxidant. Berries also have another potent compound called ellagic acid, which is as important to its beneficial effects as sulforaphane is to those of broccoli. Recent research has shown ellagic acid to be a very important chemopreventive agent because of its ability to keep DNA from harm. The results of detailed molecular studies by researchers D. Barch, Ph.D., published in *Carcinogenesis* in 1996, and B. Narayanan, Ph.D., published in *Cancer Letters* in 1999, agree that ellagic acid prevents binding of carcinogens to DNA. Beyond that, epidemiological studies have shown that eating fruits containing ellagic acid lowers the incidence of heart disease and cancer.

Ellagic acid may actually change a person's genetic predisposition to cancer. An analysis of recent medical school research shows that ellagic acid kills cervical cancer cells in particular and performs similarly on cancer cells in the breast, pancreas, esophagus, skin, colon, and prostate.

Many more studies have shown the anticancer effect of ellagic acid and its protective effect against radiation damage to chromosomes.

BLUEBERRIES

Among all fruits and vegetables, blueberries contain the highest antioxidant capability, according to the United States Department of Agriculture. Adding half a cup of fresh blueberries to your daily diet, or frozen blueberries out of season, will most likely double your antioxidant intake from food.

Blueberries' deep pigmentation comes from a class of flavonoids called anthocyanins, which often occur in nature with proanthocyanidins, another powerful antioxidant. The blueness of blueberries and the redness of strawberries and raspberries are due to this same class of compounds. Elderberry, persimmon, tart red cherries, red and purple grapes, beets, purple cabbage, and the peel of the purple eggplant also contain anthocyanins and proanthocyanidins. The high concentration of these compounds is responsible for the protective effect of blueberries against brain aging, heart disease, and cancer.

The flavonoids in blueberries raise the levels of the important antioxidant glutathione. This substance reduces inflammation in the brain, a condition thought by many experts to play a major role in Alzheimer's, Parkinson's, and other diseases of aging. Patients with Parkinson's have been known to have low levels of glutathione in their brain tissue.

Yet, perhaps the most astounding aspect of research on blueberries has been in the area of brain longevity. In research done by James Joseph, M.D., at Tufts University, rats equivalent in age to sixty-five-year-old humans were fed an amount of dried aqueous blueberry extract equal to one half cup for a person. Other experimental groups received vitamin E, dried aqueous spinach extract, or strawberry extract. After eight weeks, by which time the rats were seventy-five human years old, they took part in several tests of memory and mobility that the researchers dubbed the "rat Olympics."

All the rats showed some improvement on the memory and mobility tests. But the "blueberry rats" experienced the most dramatic improvement in balance and motor coordination. In one challenge, the blueberry rats did more than twice as well as their nearest competitors. Not only did the blueberry rats perform better than did other rats their own age, their scores indicated that they had been rejuvenated to the level of a young rat. In other words, the blueberry extract had a powerful anti-aging effect. To quote Dr. Joseph,

> This is the first study that has shown that dietary supplementation with fruit extracts that are high in phytonutrient antioxidants can actually reverse some of the age-related neuronal and behavioral dysfunction.

The significance of this statement should not go unnoticed. A half cup of blueberries a day for humans may reverse the deterioration of brain function that often occurs with aging.

BLUEBERRIES AND BRAIN LONGEVITY: THE DOPAMINE CONNECTION

In my first book, *Brain Longevity*, published in 1997, I wrote, "The brain is flesh and blood like the rest of the body." At the time, this was considered to be a revolutionary statement. Most conventional neurologists then thought that cognitive decline was a given and that nothing could be done to prevent or reverse age-related loss of mental function. It is now an accepted medical principle that many things can be done to maximize brain power in old age. Using nutrition; supplements; stress-relieving meditation; and physical, mental, and mind/body exercises, you can regenerate your mind and memory. You don't have to suffer a degenerating tumble in brain power.

Because your brain is flesh and blood like the rest of the body, it is dependent on blood flow for its rich supply of oxygen and glucose. Your brain also needs proper antioxidant protection as well as stabilization of its membrane, which tends to wear out with age just like the bottom of your tennis shoe. As we age, the stress chemical cortisol, sometimes called the death hormone, rises. Cortisol has three negative effects on your brain:

1. It reduces the ability of glucose to enter your brain cells, thereby reducing your mental energy. This decrease in energy output affects primarily the frontal lobes of the brain and an anatomical structure called the anterior cingulate gyrus.

2. When the energy drops in the frontal lobes, you cannot think well or express your personality properly. Neither can you coordinate

multiple tasks. Taken together, this array of mental abilities organized by the frontal lobes of your brain is called executive function. The cingulate gyrus also governs different attributes of cognitive function such as attention span, focus, mood, and impulse control.

3. Finally, cortisol causes a precipitous drop in your brain's level of important neurotransmitters, including acetylcholine, the memory chemical, and dopamine, the pleasure and mobility hormone. These decreases have disastrous consequences for mental function because of dopamine's numerous important physiological features.

Adequate levels of dopamine are needed for the rewards and pleasures of life such as motivation, zest, ambition, and sex drive as well as motor function and memory. A significant drop of dopamine levels in your brain leads to unhealthy aging. Scientists at Brookhaven National Laboratory used a sophisticated form of x-ray study, positron emission tomography (PET scan), in which radioactive particles are injected and then traced. Using this approach, they discovered an age-related decline in dopamine D2 receptors. Apparently, in normal aging, our dopamine level drops by approximately 6 percent each decade. This is critically important today because life span is being extended medically. What good is it to live long but not be able to concentrate, remember, or enjoy a pleasant mood?

In addition, dopamine stimulates your pituitary gland to release growth hormone, with its veritable treasure of anti-aging benefits. Dopamine also helps regulate insulin levels, which maintain the healthy metabolism that is so important for weight control. And, dopamine is important for maintaining immune function, which lessens as we age.

Dr. Joseph's research team at Tufts University found that when animals are fed blueberries they have an increased ability to manufacture and release dopamine. This correlates with a significant reversal of the motor dysfunction that occurs with aging. Although more research still needs to be done in this area, the implications are far reaching, especially when you consider that one of the most popular anti-aging medicines, deprenyl, has a very similar mode of action.

The worldwide popularity of deprenyl is due to its use in fighting degenerative brain diseases such as Parkinson's and Alzheimer's, where magnificent results have occurred. What if you could experience a similar benefit just from eating blueberries? What if by eating one half cup of blueberries a day, you could turn back the clock naturally? Well, research has shown that you may be able to do just that. What a delicious way to stay young and vital.

BILBERRIES: THE EYES HAVE IT

As you are well aware, we are experiencing a phenomenon known as global warming, which causes not only hotter temperatures but also more solar rays, or sunlight. This enhanced exposure to sunlight depletes your supply of the chemical rhodopsin, or visual purple, which is responsible for maintaining night vision. A bilberry is a small, round, dark berry. The phytonutrients found in bilberries, called anthocyanins, increase your rhodopsin, just as the anthocyanins in carrots do.

Bilberries also increase blood circulation to the retina, the large nerve in the eye. Research has shown that bilberry and vitamin E have a success rate as high as 97 percent in halting cataract progression. In another exciting study, patients given bilberries found that either their visual deterioration stabilized or their eyesight actually improved compared with a control group, whose members experienced further loss of sight.

Eyesight improvement or stabilization with the use of bilberries is yet another revolutionary finding about a fruit used as medicine. But, if you ask your ophthalmologist whether myopia is progressive, the answer will most often be "yes, you need stronger corrective lenses every year or so." Many of my healing partners have not needed stronger lenses nearly that often once they added bilberries to their diet or took them in capsule form.

CRANBERRIES

New research published in the *British Medical Journal* in 2002 confirms what many women already know: drinking cranberry juice helps treat or prevent painful urinary tract infections. This is good news, because 60 percent of women endure this ailment at some point in their lives. Research shows that women with cystitis or bladder infection reduce the chance of its recurrence within six months by half when they drink one glass of cranberry juice a day.

Cranberries, like other berries we've discussed, contain the phytonutrient ellagic acid, a potent antioxidant and cancer fighter. This substance sends very important anticancer signals to your genes, blocking both the onset of cancer and its spread. Cranberries also contain the antioxidant quercetin, which helps lower the risk of heart disease and stroke.

Quercetin sends a very positive healing signal to your genes, which also stops cancer-causing agents from injuring your DNA.

CITRUS FRUIT

Grapefruit, oranges, lemons, and limes are all rich in vitamin C and other vitamins. They also contain several important phytonutrients. Grapefruit—and especially its seed extract, which can be obtained in capsules or drops—is a powerful natural antibiotic. If you feel a cold coming on, blend one peeled grapefruit in a juicer with water, drink the liquid, and feel it work in minutes. Or buy grapefruit seed extract and put a few drops in a glass of juice. This extract is very effective in rapidly eliminating cold and flu symptoms.

Oranges contain a higher level of vitamin C than any other fruit except kiwi. However, many of the benefits of oranges to the cardiovascular and immune systems come from the fruit's vast array of phytonutrients, including terpene, and limonene, which is also found in lemons and limes. It's best to buy organic oranges. If you buy a regular orange that was picked green, you may find that drinking its juice causes joint pain or arthritis-like symptoms. This is because the citric acid in the orange has not had time to convert to fructose sugar, and it therefore has very little vitamin C. Also, some nonorganic oranges are sprayed with red dye and then waxed to look fresher and prolong shelf life. Oranges may also be sprayed with fungicides. So enjoy your oranges, but go organic.

Lemons are an excellent blood purifier and liver stimulant. At the change of seasons or if you are feeling a bit sluggish, begin your day with a glass of lemon drink. You can make it by mixing the juice of half a lemon with a glass of warm water. I strongly recommend drinking through a straw, as lemon juice can decrease your tooth enamel.

GRAPES

The health benefits of wine don't come only from the alcohol. In fact, many of the same benefits can be achieved from drinking grape juice, because grapes contain a great deal of the antioxidant quercetin and the phytonutrient resveratrol, which is found in the skins. Resveratrol thins the blood and boosts the level of HDL cholesterol, the "good" kind. Red grapes are also antibacterial and antiviral. Remember that grapes are also heavily sprayed; it is therefore best to consume organic grapes.

KIWI FRUIT

Kiwis are one of the most underrated healing foods. Not only are they incredibly high in vitamin C, containing sixteen times more than oranges, but also they contain a huge amount of vitamin E. Because of their rich array of disease-fighting antioxidants and phytonutrients, they are often prescribed in yoga nutritional therapy to help fight cancer and heart disease. I often add kiwi to my morning smoothie for its rich array of vitamins, minerals, and phytonutrients. It has a tart, yet pleasant taste.

MELONS

Cantaloupe, watermelon, honeydew, and other melons are all potent medicines as well as delicious fruit. Cantaloupes have lots of zinc, which is important for the prostate gland. Half a cantaloupe also contains more vitamins A and C than an equal amount of just about any other fruit. Cantaloupe is very high in potassium as well. I enjoy mixing one quarter of a cantaloupe with some fresh watermelon and other fruit in my juicer for a refreshing and nutritious pick-me-up. Try it in the morning or midafternoon instead of coffee or soda. The natural vitamin and mineral content of this drink will give you a lift. It also has a safe diuretic effect.

Watermelon is one of the very colorful fruits that contain high amounts of lycopene and glutathione—anticancer, antioxidant, and anti-aging phytonutrients. It's very good for detoxifying the body and can be used for a short fast that gives great pleasure. I'll never forget my first watermelon fast. I was visiting a friend in Brazil, an alternative medical doctor named Guru Dev, whose assistant came from the Amazon River basin. This chap was an outstanding herbalist and provided me with daily herbal remedies to complement my watermelon fast. I not only drank the juice but ate the fruit in chunks. After just three days I was very tuned in and meditating very deeply. As I think back, this was one of the greatest highs I have ever experienced. When I boarded the plane for home, I was definitely in an altered state. I couldn't even touch the in-flight meal. Regular foods looked and tasted like cardboard. Try a watermelon fast sometime and experience your higher self.

PEARS

You should know about pears for one special reason. In yoga nutritional therapy, they are considered to be excellent for preventing and reducing fibroid tumors and other benign growths in the body. A patient of mine had a benign tumor of the parotid gland and had to have the intruder removed by surgery. Fortunately, everything went well. A few months later, however, she developed some gynecological problems.

Because this was such a complicated case, I asked my teacher, Yogi Bhajan, for his opinion. He suggested using pears and pear juice. The patient followed the recommendation, and to this date neither her parotid nor her fibroid tumor has returned. The reason pears are so effective against lumps and bumps is thought to be its high content of the phytonutrient ellagic acid, the mineral boron, and an insoluble fiber called lignin. Together, these compounds act synergistically.

TROPICAL FRUIT

Besides being rich in phytonutrients, mango, papaya, and pineapple are also overflowing with vitamin C. Best of all, they are sweet and tasty. Mango and papaya help break down toxins in your body and, like pineapples, are rich in digestive enzymes that help you process other foods, such as proteins and carbohydrates. In addition to watermelon, I have fasted on pineapple several times. It is one food you can live on exclusively for a prolonged time because of its extraordinary nutrient content.

Pineapple can also restore enzymatic activity to a weak digestive system. Sometimes your stomach becomes weak because of stress or nervous exhaustion. When that happens, eat pineapple or drink its juice. Even better, mix a green drink powder with pineapple juice. The green drink contains many trace elements useful for optimal brain and immune function, and the pineapple juice helps you assimilate them. Pineapple is also a rich source of manganese, which helps promote bone health and strength in women. Moreover, pineapple contains bromelain, an anti-inflammatory enzyme, which makes it a wonderful fruit to help prevent and reduce the pain of arthritis and other painful conditions.

FOOD LOG EXERCISE #5

It is much easier to use the phytonutrients in berries and other fruits and vegetables as preventive medicine than to wait until a disease has been discovered. Once a person has gotten so far out of balance that cancer is present, for example, it is difficult to activate the healing force. Cancer and all other diseases represent a complex psychological, physical, and emotional imbalance. Once the diagnosis of a severe illness has been made, other factors (such as conventional medical treatment) come into play. My recommendation is to practice preventive nutritional medicine now by eating all these fruits we've discussed on a more regular basis. Don't forget to note how you feel in your food journal. If an illness does develop, your body will respond better because you will have already built a strong foundation.

FOOD LOG EXERCISE #6

If trying to remember exactly which vegetables and fruit to eat is too hard, just use this little trick: eat a rainbow as part of your daily diet.

1. **Red:** Tomatoes in any form, including sauce, juice, or sliced. Also pink grapefruit, watermelon, apples, and beets.
2. **Purple:** Grapes, peppers, prunes, plums, cherries, cranberries, raisins, and (my favorite) blueberries.
3. **Orange:** Pumpkins, carrots, winter squash, sweet potatoes, mangoes, apricots, and cantaloupes.
4. **Orange-yellow:** Oranges, orange juice, tangerines, grapefruit, peaches, lemons, limes, papaya, pineapple, and nectarines.

Excerpt from chart "Does Your Diet Include the Seven Colors of Health?" from *What Color Is Your Diet?* by David Heber, copyright 2001 by David Heber, M.D., Ph.D. Reprinted by permission of HarperCollins Publishers, Inc.

5. **Yellow-green:** Peas, beans, spinach, peppers, collard greens, cucumber, mustard greens, kiwi, and avocados.
6. **Green:** Broccoli, Brussels sprouts, cauliflower, cabbage, kale, and bok choy.
7. **White-green:** Garlic, onions, celery, leeks, asparagus, pears, artichokes, endive, mushrooms, chives, and soy.

For a new supermarket experience, try shopping by color. Follow the list above. First place red foods in your cart, then purple, and so on down the line. Put each color food in a separate part of your cart. It makes shopping a lot of fun and increases your awareness of the beautiful and healing colors of the rainbow our Creator has given us to eat.

CHAPTER 6

Beyond the Rainbow of Vegetables and Fruit

SUPER FOODS

A super food is a nutritionally dense food. That is, super foods contain concentrated amounts of vitamins, minerals, amino acids, enzymes, and other components that provide many times the power of even the most nutritious vegetables, such as broccoli. The trace elements in super foods are more easily absorbed than those in supplements, and they are therefore especially useful to people with digestive difficulties. I have prescribed super foods such as spirulina, blue-green algae, chlorella, wheatgrass, and others as part of my brain longevity program for many years and have found them to provide rapid improvement in mental energy and overall health. As a result of more than half a century of farming chemicals, American soil lacks many important nutrients. Eating an organically grown, whole foods diet, and adding super foods, means you're taking control of your nutrition.

Many conventional doctors and nutritionists are skeptical about super foods. The main reason, I believe, is their lack of experience in using them, either personally or professionally.

Super foods can be broken down into two main groups: green foods and sea vegetables. Contrary to conventional thinking, green super foods—those high in chlorophyll—are useful to the human body. Green super foods can help you to:

- Renew tissues
- Build blood
- Counteract radiation
- Improve liver health
- Purify and detoxify your body
- Clear up skin problems
- Relieve constipation
- Eliminate bad breath and body odor
- Remove drug deposits and carcinogens
- Relieve inflammation, such as arthritis

The five chief green super foods are: blue-green algae, spirulina, chlorella, barley and wheat grass, and alfalfa grass. What these five have in common is that they produce energy—something that seems to be lacking in many people today. The high concentration of essential fatty acids and vitamins in green super foods will supercharge your system. No foods are closer to nature than these miraculous micro algae healing plants.

BLUE-GREEN ALGAE

Blue-green algae is the great-great grandfather of over 30,000 different species of algae. It is very energizing because of its rich array of nutrients. Nutritionally, it is very similar to spirulina, which is actually bred in living ponds, while blue-green algae grows in the wild. Blue-green algae and the other super foods contain chlorophyll, which is similar in structure to hemoglobin, the oxygen-carrying compound in your blood. Clorophyll can help your body regenerate your blood, purify your system, and relieve the inflammation of arthritis and skin conditions. Holistic dentists use blue-green algae to help cure gingivitis.

SPIRULINA

Spirulina is an excellent fuel for the cells, increasing stamina and energy. It is so effective in increasing endurance that many long distance runners use it to improve their performance. Spirulina is a high-protein food that also contains antioxidants, minerals, and essential fatty acids. In addition to these nutrients, its health-giving properties have been attributed to chlorophyll, which is responsible for its green color. Recently, however, scientists have identified a rare emerald-green pigment unique to spirulina that may inhibit cancer.

CHLORELLA

Because chlorella contains twice the chlorophyll of other algae, it is the greenest of all the superfoods. It helps our cell walls fortify themselves against invading viruses and toxins. In addition, chlorella's rich store of cell-generating RNA and DNA helps regenerate tissues. Because of that property, I have found it quite useful in helping patients recover from surgery or a painful injury such as an inflamed shoulder. Biochemists call the unique chemical mix in chlorella controlled growth factor. It can bring about a dramatic increase in your energy and immune power.

BARLEY AND WHEAT GRASS

Throughout history, wheat and barley grass have been used for energy, blood purification, and pain relief from arthritis. These grasses have more nutrients than any other land vegetable: 92 minerals, 22 vitamins, all 8 essential amino acids, and many of the phytonutrients we have discussed. Wheat grass and barley grass have high concentrations of the anti-aging enzyme super oxide dimutase (SOD), which helps protect your cells from free radical damage.

I remember once sitting with my master and asking him about wheat grass. He told me that it is such a powerful detoxifying agent that most Americans have to be careful when drinking it because of all the meat they have consumed. I have found that to be true. Many people complain of nausea when they gulp down a shot of pure wheat grass. The cause is a rapid release of toxins in the liver. My recommendation is to either drink wheat grass slowly or mix it with water.

ALFALFA GRASS

The word *alfalfa* means "father" in Arabic. This grain has great strengthening and restorative powers. According to naturalists, it lowers blood pressure, improves digestion, and helps people with cancer have more energy, appetite, and optimism.

You can take advantage of the dense concentration of micronutrients found in green super foods by eating them separately or absorbing them together in a powdered mix such as the Longevity Green Drink (see Appendix E,

Resources). I recommend using a mix because of the vast array of nutrients it contains. For an energy-producing drink, put ¼ to ½ teaspoonful of green mix in a cup of fresh orange juice or pineapple juice, stir well, and drink. Protein powder, flaxseed oil, and a banana can be added to provide a sustained energy boost that lasts throughout the entire morning.

SEA VEGETABLES

Sea vegetables grow in the oceans, where they absorb fifty-six different minerals and trace elements. They provide ten times the mineral content of broccoli. Kelp contains more minerals than any other vegetable in the world. Sea vegetables are an underwater treasure. The main sea vegetables are these:

AGAR

Agar is a clear, tasteless sea vegetable that is useful in the modern kitchen. Cooked agar is an alternative to regular gelatin, which is made from the hooves of cows, horses, and pigs. Medicinally, it is a tonic to the gastrointestinal tract.

ARAME

Arame is rich in calcium, iron, and vitamins A and B. It can help keep your blood pressure under control, heal the spleen and pancreas, and help correct female hormone imbalance. Because of its rich supply of iodine, arame also benefits the thyroid.

DULSE

Dulse is especially good for women, offering more iron than any other sea vegetable.

HIZIKI

In Japanese, hiziki translates as "bearer of wealth and beauty." Ounce for ounce, it has fourteen times more calcium than milk. It builds strong bones and also soothes the nerves.

KELP

No other food contains more iodine, the mineral that helps your thyroid regulate your metabolism and weight, than kelp. Kelp also helps carry radioactive substances and heavy metals safely out of your body.

KOMBU

Kombu contains sitosterol, a chemical that helps prevent your digestive tract from absorbing cholesterol.

NORI

Nori, the jade-green ribbon that is wrapped around sushi, is higher in protein than any other sea vegetable and has more vitamin A than carrots.

WAKAME/ALARIA

Wakame is from Japan, and alaria is obtained off American coasts. They both have a very high calcium content. Wakame is used to restore energy after childbirth, illness, or surgery. It can also be enjoyed as an energizer when cooked in miso soup.

Brown sea vegetables such as kombu, arame, and hiziki all contain alginic acid. This nutrient binds to radioactive wastes and heavy metals to increase their removal from your body. Eating seaweed can help eliminate 50 to 80 percent of these toxins. The benefits of sea vegetables probably help explain the excellent fitness and longevity enjoyed by the people of Japan. As a bonus, sea vegetables can help make you beautiful—they are good for the skin and may even help slow the balding process.

If sea vegetables are new to you, I suggest you start slowly by enjoying them at a Japanese restaurant. Then you can try the milder-tasting arame, dulse, or nori at home. You can find them in health food stores and even some conventional supermarkets. Nori is especially flavorful when combined with miso soup. Eat only a little at first, so your digestive system can adjust to the new flavors and effects of seaweed.

FLAXSEEDS AND FLAXSEED OIL

Fat in and of itself is not bad for you, but the wrong fats can damage your arteries, brain cells, and genes. The best fats are of the omega-3 type, found in certain fish such as salmon, and also in algae, olive oil, flax, and flaxseed oil. The essential fatty acids (those your body can't make) found in flax are like medicine to your cell membranes and actually boost resistance to allergens and illness. Flax can lower cholesterol, relieve arthritis, help treat multiple sclerosis, and help balance estrogen during menopause.

Many leading researchers and clinicians report that an unhealthy excess of omega-6 oils (those found in alarm foods) over omega-3 oils in the diet can cause illness. A healthful balance of omega-6 and omega-3 oils is essential to your well-being because of their role in the proper synthesis of prostaglandin hormones. Prostaglandins derived from too many omega-6 fatty acids send negative messages throughout your body: They promote incorrect cell proliferation, inflammation, and blood clotting. A proper ratio of omega-3 and omega-6 oils changes that negative message into a positive one.

Since I am a vegetarian and don't eat fish, I would be deficient in omega-3 if we didn't keep flaxseed oil in our refrigerator and use it on salads. You can also buy the seeds themselves and grind them up in a coffee grinder, then sprinkle the nutty-tasting powder over salads, baked potatoes, cereals, or popcorn.

Of course, we do need some omega-6 oils to keep our body balanced as it should be. You can get them from meat, but a far healthier source is found in beans, which are rich in omega-6 oils. Nuts also contain omega-6, and walnuts have the highest concentration.

Other nonanimal sources of "good fat" are black currant oil and evening primrose oil. They are useful against all diseases associated with inflammation, including arthritis, neurological disorders, heart disease, and disorders associated with menopause.

MUSHROOMS

Three types of mushrooms have a powerful effect on the health of the immune system: maitake, shiitake, and reishi. All three act as medicine.

MAITAKE

Maitake mushrooms have a beneficial effect on cardiovascular health and diabetes, in addition to having an anticancer effect. It is believed that their anticancer and immune-enhancing effects are related to their content of polysaccharides—sugarlike molecules that are structural components of many cells. Polysaccharides stimulate our roving immune system cells, called macrophages, to begin a cascade of immune-enhancing events. These events lead to an increase in natural killer cell activity, which destroys malignant cells in the body.

According to several published reports, maitake mushrooms work to increase the effectiveness of conventional cancer therapy, thus allowing for a lower effective dose of cancer-fighting drugs. They also lower blood pressure and help regulate blood glucose.

I suggest eating maitake mushrooms, or taking them in supplemental form, to patients with any immune deficiency disease. These include cancer, chronic fatigue syndrome, AIDS, chronic hepatitis, and environmental illness.

SHIITAKE

Shiitake mushrooms contain the phytonutrient lenitan, which is a biological response modifier that boosts the function of tumor-fighting interleukin-1, and cancer cell killers known as T lymphocytes. Many leading integrative cancer therapists prescribe shiitake mushrooms to prevent the development of cancer and stop it from spreading. Some Japanese studies show that these mushrooms may also lower cholesterol.

REISHI

Reishi mushrooms have a very high level of antioxidant activity, thanks to their content of the phytonutrient ganoderic acid. For that reason, they are considered to be a superior component of yoga nutritional therapy. I recommend eating reishi mushrooms in combination with maitake and shiitake mushrooms. When they are enjoyed together, you receive all the antioxidant, cardiovascular, and other health benefits of the three mushroom super foods at the same time.

TEA

Tea, especially green tea, has proven medical benefits. Just like fruits and vegetables, green tea contains generous amounts of phytonutrients. In this instance, the phytonutrient responsible for the cancer-fighting and heart-protecting qualities of green tea is epigallocatechin gallate (EGCG). In scientific studies, EGCG has shown impressive activity against many kinds of cancer. Ideally, you need about four cups of green tea a day to get the benefits, but because you'll be eating many different synergistic foods as medicine, any amount you drink is a help. I actually recommend fewer than four cups of green tea daily because, although it contains less caffeine than coffee or black tea, it is still a stimulating beverage. My feeling is that we need less stimulation, not more. You can safely drink four cups of decaffeinated green tea daily and still enjoy its many health benefits.

Another tea I've found refreshing and salubrious is yerba mate, from South America. It is a naturally stimulating herbal energy tea that doesn't produce a letdown. Yerba mate induces mental clarity, sustains energy levels, and improves mood. It also has been reported to boost immunity, relieve allergies, aid weight loss, and increase libido. The effect of one cup in the morning usually lasts all day. I particularly find it useful when fasting. You can find it at most health food stores.

GRAINS, SPROUTS, SEEDS, NUTS, AND BEANS

One of my early mentors in holistic medicine was the late Paavo Airola, Ph.D. Dr. Airola was from Eastern Europe and was one of the original pioneers in using food as medicine. When I first met him, I was struck by his prescription for a long and healthy life. Dr. Airola suggested that the staples of the human diet should be seeds, nuts, and especially grains. I find that many writers on nutritional topics—and also physicians—don't quite understand the proper use of grains. They want you to eat too much, which can lead to obesity. Dr. Airola saw grains as necessary but cautioned that they should be eaten in moderation. For example, his millet stew would contain ¼ cup of cooked millet with a generous helping of steamed vegetables, including carrots, cabbage, cauliflower, and perhaps some kale or broccoli. He also favored brown rice, oats, barley, buckwheat, amaranth, bulgur, corn, kamut, quinoa, and a small amount of wheat. He studied longevity and health all around the world and found that many long-lived people, especially those in a certain section in Romania, ate grains as a staple of their diet.

Grains not only are an excellent source of protein but also are very high in fiber, many vitamins and minerals, and unsaturated fatty acids, which are indispensable for maximal health. Moreover, grains have a high content of natural vitamin E, which many research studies reveal is critically important to prevent premature aging of the immune, cardiovascular, and nervous systems. Grains are also nature's best source of the B-complex vitamins.

Dr. Airola also touted the very healthful benefits of eating sprouts. A sprout is a baby plant as it begins to grow from its seed. Because the sprout is a living food, it has a very high nutritional value. It is also easy to digest. Wheatberries, mung beans, alfalfa seeds, sunflower seeds, lentils, and soybeans can all be sprouted to optimize your nutrition—and, of course, I've already turned you into an expert on the benefits of broccoli sprouts. Sprouts can be eaten raw in salads, stir-fried, or even blended in a smoothie.

According to Dr. Airola's research, with which I agree, all seeds and nuts should be eaten raw. Those that can be sprouted or bought sprouted, such as alfalfa sprouts, wheat sprouts, or broccoli sprouts, should be used in that form whenever possible. Sunflower seeds, pumpkin seeds, almonds, peanuts, sesame seeds, buckwheat, and soybeans all contain complete proteins; therefore, their nutritional value is complete without further preparation.

All kinds of beans are very high in protein. There are several advantages to getting your protein from beans. One reason is that beans are easier on your budget than animal sources of protein. But beyond that, they are less likely to contain high concentrations of environmental pollutants. Also, they do not send alarm signals to your cells, and hence your genes, because beans are devoid of saturated fat—the kind found in meat. Finally, because the protein found in beans is less concentrated than that found in meat, you can have a bit more protein in your diet without taking the chance of stressing your system.

SOY

The answer to every human illness can be found in nature. In Japan, where soy is consumed as a staple, the incidence of prostate cancer is 18 percent of what it is in the United States, where most people haven't yet made the transition to a high-protein, low-fat diet. In Okinawa, where the people consume even more soy protein than those in Japan, not only do the natives suffer less chronic debilitating disease, they are the longest-lived people in the world. It is also important to point out that Okinawans consume approximately 30 percent fewer total calories than those living on mainland Japan. As you recall, lower caloric intake equals longer life.

The primary reason soy is such an excellent medical food is that it contains two isoflavones: genestein and daidzein. Both are well known for their regenerative and disease-preventive qualities. Isoflavones are part of a class of compounds called phytoestrogens, which are weaker versions of the estrogen that is produced naturally by women. Isoflavones appear to help prevent disease by blocking the negative effects of natural estrogen. In his book *Soya for Health,* Stephen Holt, M.D., presents over a thousand references on the multiple benefits of soy for developing and maintaining maximum health. Among soy's documented advantages are these:

- Reduction in the risk of heart disease
- Protection against breast cancer
- Reduction in the risk of prostate cancer
- A decrease in symptoms of menopause
- Stronger bones and prevention of osteoporosis

Soy is available today as tofu in the famous white blocks found in most food stores, as well as in many meatless items such as soy burgers. The creative minds in the natural food industry have also recently invented other ways to enjoy this food. Soy hot dogs and other meat substitutes, for example, are found in every health food store (see Appendix C).

FOOD LOG EXERCISE #7

Explore your conventional supermarket or health food store and discover some of the foods I've discussed in this chapter, such as spirulina, arame, flaxseed, shiitake mushrooms, millet, alfalfa sprouts, pumpkin seeds, almonds, and lentils. If you are unfamiliar with soy, look for it as well. Then choose a recipe from below, and let your palate become familiar with these foods. Enjoy!

Millet Loaf
Makes 8 servings

2 cups millet
6 cups water

¼–½ cup grated ginger
1 teaspoon sea salt
1 tablespoon cumin powder
1 teaspoon oregano
1 tablespoon caraway seeds
1 teaspoon tarragon
1 teaspoon parsley
2 large white onions, finely chopped
5 cloves garlic, minced
2 stalks celery, finely chopped
1–2 tablespoons Braggs Liquid Aminos

Preheat oven to 375°F. Combine millet, water, ginger, salt, *half* the cumin, and the other spices in a saucepan, and simmer on low for 45 minutes or until liquid is absorbed. Stir occasionally. Add onions, garlic, and celery to millet, together with Braggs Liquid Aminos. Millet should be soft and mushy (add more water if not). Spread in a deep baking pan. Sprinkle the top with remaining cumin, and bake covered for at least 45 minutes or until crispy on top. Try it with mushroom gravy.

Mushroom Gravy
Makes 2½ cups

2 large white onions, sliced
1 teaspoon extra virgin olive oil
1 teaspoon tarragon
1 teaspoon basil
1 teaspoon parsley
Approximately 1 cup pure water
3–4 tablespoons Braggs Liquid Aminos
4 fresh shiitake mushrooms
4 white mushrooms
2 portobello mushrooms
2 cloves garlic

2 tablespoons water
1 tablespoon cornstarch or arrowroot

Sauté onions in olive oil. Add tarragon, basil, and parsley. Add 1 cup of water, and continue sautéing over medium heat for approximately 25 minutes until onions are translucent and caramelized. Add more water and Braggs Liquid Aminos when needed to keep from sticking.

While onions cook, discard mushroom stems and chop mushroom caps into small slices, and finely chop garlic. Once onions are cooked thoroughly, add mushrooms and garlic, and continue to sauté for approximately 5 more minutes. In a separate bowl, mix 2 tablespoons water with cornstarch or arrowroot, then stir in mixture with mushrooms and onions, and cook to thicken—about 2 minutes. Serve over millet loaf.

Millet Stew
Makes 4 servings

3½ cups water
1 cup millet, rinsed
⅓ cup quinoa
1 white onion, chopped
2 cloves garlic, minced
½ inch ginger, grated
½ teaspoon oregano
½ teaspoon basil
¼ teaspoon sage
½ teaspoon sea salt
1 tablespoon Braggs Liquid Aminos

Combine all ingredients in a covered saucepan and simmer on low for 45 minutes, or until millet balls have broken up and all the water is absorbed. Do not stir while cooking. If millet is not soft, you may need to add up to ½ cup of hot water and cook for another 10 minutes.

Tofu-Veggie Combo
Makes 4 servings

1 white onion, chopped
2 cloves garlic, minced
3 teaspoons extra virgin olive oil
½ bunch asparagus, chopped
2 large carrots, chopped
1 cup peas
1 large tomato, chopped
1 package Mori-Nu light firm tofu
1½ teaspoons zattar (herb mix from Middle Eastern stores)
½ teaspoon crushed red chili

Place onion, garlic, and olive oil in a pan, and sauté over medium heat until onion is softened (about 2 minutes). Add asparagus, carrots, peas, and tomato. Let simmer for five minutes.

In the meantime, drain the tofu and cut it into chunks. After 5 minutes, add the tofu, zattar, and red chili, and simmer for another 5 to 7 minutes, stirring often to prevent sticking.

CHAPTER 7

From Pyramids to Principles

The pyramid is a pretty good invention—something we've known since the time of ancient Egypt. In the past fifty years or so, the pyramid has gotten lots of use as a means of teaching people the healthiest way to eat. The shape allows us to illustrate the amounts we need of different kinds of foods in our diet.

USDA PYRAMID

The United States Department of Agriculture (USDA) published the original dietary pyramid and its successors. The latest one, dating from the 1980s, emphasizes the importance of maintaining a healthy weight, choosing a diet low in fat and cholesterol, using salt and sodium in moderation, and eating a variety of foods. It is a good starting point, but because of its overly simplistic approach, it has become very outdated.

As you examine the pyramid (see figure), you can see that the base consists of processed carbohydrates such as breads, cereals, rice, and pasta, with no mention of the type of grain—whole grain, white flour, or other—of which they should consist. This is a great mistake, because white flour products, which are the most popular in the United States, are all low-fiber foods that can contribute to obesity.

Vegetables and fruits are divided into two groups on the next tier of the pyramid. This lessens their importance in comparison with processed and perhaps refined carbohydrates. According to David Heber, M.D., Ph.D., the director of the UCLA Center for Human Nutrition and author of *What Color Is*

U.S.D.A. FOOD GUIDE PYRAMID

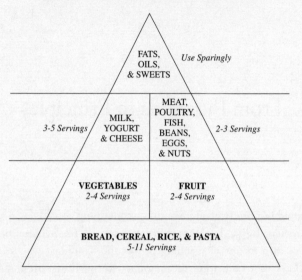

Your Diet, this was done "because it was felt by some committee members that it would be wrong to combine them, since fruits taste better than vegetables and would probably be overemphasized in the consumer's food choices." However, the real-life problem is that not enough of either of them is eaten.

A dairy group consisting of milk, yogurt, and cheeses (all high in saturated fat) is featured side by side with meats, nuts, and beans in the next tier of the pyramid. This combination was expected to increase the consumption of dairy and hence calcium. However, the scientists were completely wrong in their assumption that calcium could be obtained only by eating dairy.

Dots of sugar and oil sit atop the pyramid, implying that these nonfoods are an important part of the all-American diet. They are not.

The USDA pyramid is, regrettably, a prescription for obesity and poor health. As such, new dietary pyramids have popped up, including the Mediterranean diet pyramid and, most recently, the California cuisine pyramid.

MEDITERRANEAN DIET PYRAMID

The Mediterranean diet pyramid moves us closer to an ideal mix of foods for good health and longevity. It emphasizes olive oil and fish over meat, and cheese over milk. Walter Willett, Ph.D., of Harvard University, the creator of this pyramid, was the first scientist who urged us to pay attention to the type of fat we eat rather than just the amount. Although the Mediterranean diet pyramid does not insist that we cut our total intake of fat, it does by design emphasize good fat, the omega-3s, which are found in fish and olive oil. As you can see, fresh fruits and vegetables are in a more prominent position than in the USDA pyramid and also are given greater importance than red meat, which is to be eaten sparingly.

MEDITERRANEAN DIET PYRAMID

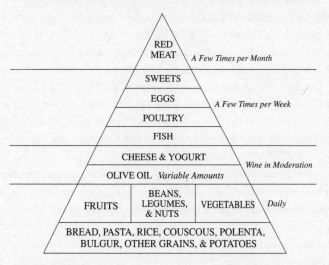

There is a large amount of good scientific evidence to support the Mediterranean diet. The most often quoted example is the Lyon heart study, which randomly assigned three hundred cardiac patients to a Mediterranean-style diet and a similar number to an American Heart Association (AHA)-style diet. Recall that the Mediterranean diet emphasizes a rich array of phytonutrients and olive oil, whereas the AHA diet uses polyunsaturated fats. After twenty-seven months, the study was stopped for ethical reasons because the group consuming the Mediterranean diet had 70 percent fewer heart attacks. After four years, the people who continued with a Mediterranean diet had an even more pronounced advantage, enjoying a 61 percent lower rate of cancer and a 56 percent lower overall mortality rate.

More than cold, hard science supports eating in this way. I am married to an Italian woman from Rome. My wife, Kirti, has been in the United States for ten years. Because I have been lucky enough to visit her family in Italy many times, I can tell you the realities of the Mediterranean diet as it is lived. First of all, it's a lot healthier than you can sense from the pyramid. At home, Italians eat very well. The food is fresh, often grown in "la mamma's" garden. The pasta, which can be eaten often (twice daily) to seldom (twice weekly), is also fresh and, most importantly, not made from overly processed grain.

For some reason I never ate pasta growing up. So the first time I went to Kirti's home and ate it there, it was a revelation. I felt as if I were in heaven. It was cooked al dente, in stark contrast to the limp noodles you so often get in an Italian restaurant here in the States. Moreover, the pasta there is rarely a main course. It is usually served first, followed by a large fresh salad with a light olive oil dressing. Then comes the protein—perhaps a small piece of meat or fish, or sometimes a delicious assortment of cheese. On the table at this time is also placed a selection of fresh vegetables, such as spinach, other greens, or eggplant. For dessert, a bowl of fresh fruit is placed on the table. My brother-in-law, Cesare, may take an apple; my sister-in law, Virginia, may choose a beautiful bunch of fresh red grapes.

There are actually three more things to discuss when we consider the Mediterranean diet: wine, fun, and exercise. Everyone seems to make a big deal about the wine in the Mediterranean diet, but I must tell you that only a small amount of it is actually consumed. Moreover, in my experience, what is drunk is commonly diluted with water. In other words, the wine is more for digestion than for its effect on consciousness—although I'm sure the latter is part of the relaxing attitude of the Mediterranean meal. Scientifically speaking, red wine is healthful because it contains resveratrol, an effective cancer-preventive compound. It actually inhibits tumor development activity in DNA. In yoga nutritional therapy, drinking wine is optional for two reasons. First, you can obtain the same resveratrol benefits from eating grapes, drinking grape juice, or taking grapeseed extract supplements. That is important to many of my patients because they've discovered that regular alcohol consumption makes it harder to meditate. Second, blood thinning, an important medicinal effect of wine, can be obtained from omega-3 oils and certain supplements such as ginkgo. Of course, if you are taking anticoagulants for heart disease or another illness, please consult your doctor before using wine or nutrients for their blood-thinning effect.

In addition, I have come to realize that the healthfulness of the Mediterranean diet comes just as much from the socializing and family fun as it does from the excellent array of phytonutrients on the table. Lively conversation, fooling around, and good old family interaction always characterize Italian mealtimes. It is community spirit at its best. More often than not, a long walk follows the meal, rather than plopping down on the couch to watch television. I think it all came together for me when my son, Sat, said something after a particularly wonderful meal. This feast featured his favorite pasta made by my mother-in law, Paola, with one of the family's prized recipes. "Hey, Dad," Sat said dreamily. "I think this food has psychoactive properties." And it does. You simply feel great after eating a true Mediterranean meal.

CALIFORNIA CUISINE PYRAMID

As you've learned, fruits and vegetables protect your DNA by counteracting the inflammation process, increasing antioxidant activity, and reducing the consumption of bad fats and refined sugars. But as Dr. Heber mentioned, this is not enough. He feels that herbs and spices such as garlic, chilies, and other taste enhancers should have their own specific section. To accomplish this, he devised his own pyramid, the California cuisine pyramid, in 1997. This pyramid has fruits and vegetables at the base to encourage the adequate intake of phytonutrients in foods that are low in calories. As you can see, high-fiber whole cereals and grains occupy the next tier. The third tier encourages adequate intake of protein and the avoidance of extra fats and calories. The top of the pyramid includes nuts, seeds, oil, cheese, and spices rather than the drops of oil and sugar found at the top of the USDA pyramid.

Dr. Heber says, "While we can't turn back the clock to prehistoric Africa, when our genes were more perfectly adapted to a biodiverse plant environment, perhaps we can use our modern understanding of genetics to develop a better contemporary diet—one that is matched to our genes rather than to historical events and economics."

FROM PYRAMIDS TO PRINCIPLES

I agree with Dr. Heber that it is time to develop a contemporary diet. But I don't believe the answer is found in a pyramid, even in his highly enlightened

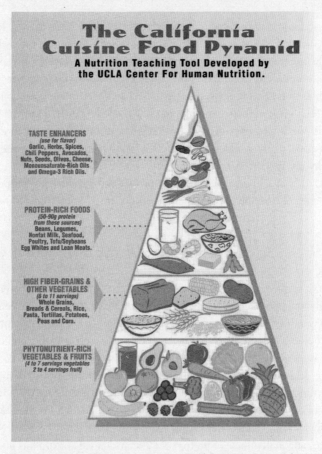

© Dr. David Heber, *The Resolution Diet,* Avery Publishing Group, New York, 1999

one. As I mentioned in chapter 1, now is the time to move forward into Aquarian Age nutrition, which is based on yoga nutritional therapy. To do that successfully you don't need a pyramid. All you need is a basic set of principles that takes into consideration not only the need to eat well for health, but also the delicate balance between our own health and that of the environment. We must also realize that to live a strong, healthy life in this time of great challenge demands paying attention to spiritual consciousness. Now, more than ever before, we must be fit in our body, mind, and soul.

The seven principles of yoga nutritional therapy help you to restore balance to your body, mind, and spirit. They also help heal our planet. The seven principles are these:

1. Detoxify your body
2. Go organic
3. Limit or eliminate genetically engineered foods
4. Eat clean protein
5. Discover juicing and supplements
6. Cook consciously and eat mindfully
7. Make the transition to the yoga nutritional therapy diet

FOOD LOG EXERCISE #8

I know that if you begin to follow these seven principles of yoga nutritional therapy instead of relying on outdated pyramids, you will soon experience tremendous benefits. Feel free to adapt these principles to your lifestyle and preferences, so long as you heed them well. My suggestion is that you read and study the information in the next chapters at a relaxed pace. Afterward, experiment to see what suits your needs. You will soon find the missing piece of your health plan for which you have been searching.

CHAPTER 8

The First Principle: Detoxify Your Body with Colon Therapy and Fasting

Many advanced practitioners of the healing arts believe that all disease begins in the colon. Their core hypothesis is that years of inadequate bowel movements lead to toxic buildup in the small and large intestines. This sludge, as they refer to it, inhibits proper absorption of the nutritional products of digestion. Moreover, these toxins may be absorbed into the bloodstream through the multitude of gastrointestinal blood vessels, and then cause symptoms such as pain, fatigue, constipation, arthritis, gynecological problems, prostate swelling, and even cancer. While I am not convinced that all disease begins in the colon, I do agree 100 percent that toxic buildup in the bowels causes serious problems in many people.

Obviously, there must be a problem with elimination in the United States. As a nation we spend $400 million a year on three hundred-plus different brands of laxatives. The next time you go into your drugstore, visit the laxative section. You'll see it takes up five shelves and spans a good hundred feet in length. According to Vernon Cook, L.M.T., a colon health specialist, "Our cells need oxygen and nutrition. But when water is added to the white flour, cheese, sugar, meat, and other processed foods consumed by many Americans, the colon becomes coated and plugged. This inhibits the absorption of nutrients and deprives our cells of oxygen and nutrients."

Toxins that can be absorbed into our bodies through the colon must eventually lodge somewhere inside us. Let's say some of these toxins settle into your joints. One day you wake up with a pain in your wrist. The doctor diagnoses arthritis. What's the first thing he or she is likely to do? Give you a pain pill. The symptom may abate for a while, but the toxins continue to build up. The result is more pain, which sends you back to the doctor for stronger pills.

Back at the drugstore, right next to the laxative aisle, is the pain pill section, equally vast and well stocked. Are you beginning to see how all this adds up?

Additionally, according to Vernon Cook and others, when the colon remains full from lack of adequate emptying over the years, it can become prolapsed—that is, dropped. The additional weight of so much waste simply causes the colon to sag. When that happens to women, it can put pressure on the reproductive organs, causing pain and inflammation, so they seek gynecological care. Often the specialist is unaware of how improper colon health can affect other organs, and so surgery may be mistakenly recommended. It is common knowledge that many questionable operations are performed for misdiagnosed gynecological conditions every year. Although the cause of the pain is unknown, a diagnosis of fibroids may be made, and the patient is subjected to surgery with all of its attendant risks. My suggestion is that before any woman has this nonemergency surgery, she try a detoxifying fast and a colon-cleansing program.

There are misconceptions about what constitutes normal bowel movements. Conventional medical texts state that each person has his or her own normal routine, and if someone goes every three days or so, it might be all right. That is utter and complete nonsense, not backed by any science whatsoever. Ideally, you should empty your colon after every meal—that is, three times a day. You read correctly. What goes in should go out. Stools should be at least six inches long and about one half inch in diameter.

Maintaining this routine is a challenge in today's world, I know. The problem takes us back to our stressful lifestyles and overabundance of alarm foods, all of which are markedly low in fiber, without which there can be no good elimination. I recall very clearly giving anesthesia to a medical colleague for cancer surgery several years ago. He was sixty-five when he was diagnosed with colon cancer. As I read his medical history on the chart I was staggered to see that he had bowel movements only once every ten days. This has remained engraved in my memory and made me a believer in the importance of colon health to overall well-being and longevity.

For all these reasons, tissue cleansing through bowel management assumes a great importance in my medical practice and in my recommendation for fasting.

HISTORY OF COLON THERAPY

Colon therapy is an ancient form of medical treatment, having been recorded as early as 1500 B.C. in the Ebers Papyrus, an Egyptian scientific document. Until the past sixty years or so, colon therapy was an accepted and popular means for reversing the onset of illness. Today, with the increasing desire among many people to return to more natural healing, and with the development of sophisticated colonic irrigation machines, it is returning to popularity. As many as two thousand colon therapists are presently practicing in the United States.

Colonic irrigation breaks down and eliminates the impacted fecal material in the intestines. Many patients who undergo a colon cleansing release seven to ten pounds of waste and then feel much better. You can imagine how good you'd feel after getting rid of such a weight.

Colonic irrigation is simply an enema given by a professional colon hygienist, using a machine designed for this purpose. The procedure is not as uncomfortable as you might think. In my research I have found only a handful of people who felt the benefits weren't worth the nuisance of the procedure. During a colonic irrigation, water is introduced into the colon and circulates via a dual-flow tube, so no pressure is built up inside the body.

In 2000, a survey of physicians using colon therapy in their medical practices was published that verified its value. Surgeons, cancer therapists, and stomach specialists were among the doctors recommending colon therapy in the study, as reported in the November 2000 issue of the *Journal of Colon Hydrotherapy*.

FASTING FOR COLON HEALTH

The goal of a revitalization program is to cleanse your body and help activate your natural healing force. Fasting one day a week, every week of your life, can become your key to absolutely fantastic health. Remember that the human gastrointestinal system is like an elastic pipe. Unless your diet has been superb for most of your life and your elimination excellent, your food has never been entirely digested and the resultant waste completely eliminated. This pipe system traps waste, and toxins may be absorbed as a result. Fasting and tissue cleansing through bowel management will help you eliminate this foundation for illness.

All my personal experience with fasting has been positive. I have found great mental clarity and increased energy and rejuvenation in a body empty of food yet full of health and spirit. In patients, I have noted many benefits from fasting, including a decrease in arthritis symptoms, a reduction in cholesterol, lowering of high blood pressure, regression of cancer, and, of course, weight loss.

In studying case histories and interviewing many guests at one of America's most successful retreats for fasting, We Care Holistic Spa in Desert Springs, California, I have discovered that many people get their weight under control by fasting and then keep it down by following a yoga nutritional therapy program once they go home.

Fasting is effective because it allows the energy you use for digestive purposes to go toward healing and restoring balance to your body. If you give yourself a break from assimilating food, the vital force within you becomes activated. When this energy is not exhausted by the task of digesting processed alarm foods, it is ready to heal.

Here is a summary of the benefits from fasting:

- During a fast the body rids itself of damaged, diseased, aged, and dead cells.
- The building of new, healthy cells is speeded up.
- The capacity of the lungs, liver, kidneys, and skin is greatly increased, and masses of wastes and toxins are eliminated.
- Fasting allows digestive, assimilative, and protective organs to rest.
- Fasting exerts normalizing, stabilizing, and rejuvenating effects on vital physiological and mental functions.
- Fasting normalizes your relationship with food.

In our society we are inundated with unhealthy advertising messages. Next time you turn on the television, notice all the garbage that is being promoted. We are urged to eat high-sugar, low-fiber, and high-fat junk food. When was the last time you saw a fancy commercial for broccoli or blueberries? Moreover, if you drive down any major American street, you will see one fast food place after the other—glossy structures trying to convince you to eat a fatty burger, some greasy fries that long ago stopped being a potato, a doughnut and coffee, or a cola drink with enough sugar to sweeten Afghanistan and enough caffeine to fuel a medical student for a month. There is also an abundance of so-called roast beef; fried, artificially raised chicken; and synthetic pizza. No wonder we are the fattest nation in the world and have the highest incidence of degenerative disease.

Fasting completely increases your food awareness. When you fast, you will see all the unhealthy advertising messages for junk food for what they really are.

SOME IMPORTANT FASTING TIPS

There are important dos and don'ts that go along with a fasting program. While fasting, you should remove the morbid matter from your intestines by using colon therapy. If that really isn't for you, why not try an enema? Using one a day for a few days will have no negative consequences and is not addicting to your intestines, despite what misinformation you may have heard. If that doesn't appeal to you, take two 450-mg aloe vera tablets or some other natural laxative at night. You should begin the cleansing process by the next day.

As a rule, a fast is a good time to stop taking vitamin supplements. There are a few exceptions. If you have a heart condition, you can continue taking your coenzyme Q10 and vitamin E. If you are ill or immune deficient, take up to 3,000 mg of vitamin C a day with diluted fruit juice. An effervescent form of it, such as Emergen-C, is my choice. If you are very weak, take a teaspoonful of pure honey as a sweetener in your ginger or yogi spice tea.

In the beginning stages of fasting, do not stop taking your prescription medications. If you are embarking on a program to eliminate some of these medicines, make sure you discuss this with a knowledgeable physician, and try to have your fast medically supervised.

A good way to get ready for the fast is to concentrate on eating primarily steamed vegetables for a few days before you actually begin. It is also best to cut down on tobacco, alcohol, and coffee in the three or four days preceding your fast. And although this will seem obvious, it is important to remember that you are not to smoke or drink alcohol or caffeine during the fast. In fact, fasting is an outstanding, clinically proven method for rapidly and painlessly eliminating cravings for cigarettes, alcohol, and other drugs. Finally, use only fresh organic juices for your fast, and prepare them immediately before you drink them.

FREQUENTLY ASKED QUESTIONS ABOUT FASTING

1. **How do I prepare for the fast?** Eat only fruits, vegetables, and juice for three days before your fast. Cut down on caffeine, alcohol, and tobacco.

2. **Are there any contraindications to fasting?** In general, patients with severe diabetes, active infections, mental instability, weak heart, or certain types of advanced cancer should not fast. Also, fasting is not advised for pregnant women and children under the age of sixteen. Always check with your physician if you are ill and wish to fast.

3. **Can I exercise when I fast?** Yes. Walking in fresh air is excellent, as is yoga. Strenuous exercise such as extended jogging and heavy weight training should be avoided. Light exercise is crucial to help your body cleanse the blood and tissues. This is also a good time to sleep with the windows open if possible, and do a bit of sunbathing.

4. **Should I stop working while I fast?** On the contrary, you will enjoy your work more because your energy will be high. You may gain enhanced insight into a problem and solve it during a fast. This may not apply if your work requires physical labor; in that instance, I would suggest that you fast on the weekend.

5. **Will I feel hungry when I fast?** Yes, naturally, at first—but not horribly so. If you extend your fast or attend a fasting retreat, your hunger will leave you after two or three days. After that, amazingly, the longer you fast the less hungry you will feel. When your body completes the cleansing work of the fast, hunger will return. This is a reliable sign that it is time to break your fast.

HOW TO FAST

The most convenient way to fast doesn't even require total abstinence from food. Neither does it mean that you only drink water, which is a powerful way to go but not very comfortable. The fast at We Care, which can be as short as three days but typically lasts a week (and in some cases longer), involves a specific regimen of pure water, herbal teas, energy supplements, minerals, fresh organic mixed vegetable juice, and a delicious soup made from a diluted puree of steamed vegetables. During the fast, no solid food is taken, but liquids are given in great abundance. Hunger may be present for the first day or so, but then it usually vanishes as physical, mental, and spiritual energy increases.

THE THIRTY-SIX-HOUR FAST

A modified thirty-six-hour fast is a safe and sensible start to cleansing your system. This light fast will not interrupt your normal life, even if you work in an office. My good friend Joseph DeNucci, general manager of Miraval, undertakes this one-day cleanse often and has plenty of energy and clarity to handle his many responsibilities. Miraval is a destination spa—a place to go to relax, exercise, meditate, eat healthy food, learn to be in the moment, and rejuvenate your body, mind, and spirit.

On rising

Drink a cup of hot water with the juice of half a lemon. Allow one hour before breakfast. This is an excellent time for your personal spiritual practice of kundalini or other yoga, meditation, and prayer.

Breakfast

Have fresh, organic fruit and low-fat organic cottage cheese or yogurt with a very small amount of pure organic honey (optional) and 1 tablespoon of wheat germ. Drink a cup of ginger tea from the Yogi Tea company. You can find various blends of Yogi Tea in your health food store and even in some regular supermarkets. If you are so inclined, you can brew your own batch of special yogi spice tea (different from ginger tea), which is part of Hari's perfect plate (see page 137). To sweeten your tea, use fructose, stevia, or a very small amount of honey. No artificial sweeteners of any kind, and no sugar.

Lunch

Have a large green salad with raw, organic vegetables and sprouts but no meat, cheese, chicken, or fish. Do not use salad dressing that contains sugar, cheese, chemical preservatives, or monosodium glutamate (MSG). Pure virgin olive oil or flaxseed oil with a cider vinegar or lemon, fresh garlic, and herbs such as basil and tarragon make the best dressing. In place of salt, you may add a few squirts of Braggs Liquid Aminos for flavor. A slice of whole-grain or nine-grain bread with no butter can be eaten with the salad. Drink another cup of ginger tea or special yogi spice tea.

Drink at least eight glasses of pure water during the day.

Dinner

At dinner, begin your fast. Instead of eating, drink only a cup of hot water with lemon and a cup of ginger tea or yogi spice tea without honey. Drink a glass of water or two throughout the evening. Relax, read, meditate, pray, or go to sleep early. Do not watch television. Do not think much, and try not to worry. Practice being at peace with yourself and your surroundings. A nice affirmation to do as you get ready for bed (perhaps by taking a relaxing hot bath) was taught to me by Louise L. Hay, D.D.:

> I Love Myself,
> Accept Myself,
> and Appreciate Myself
> As I Am, Right Now.
> All Is Well in My World,
> And I'm at Peace.

On rising

Take your morning shower, and have a glass of warm water with lemon. Continue with your morning ritual of yoga, meditation, and prayer.

Breakfast

Have another cup of hot water with lemon and a cup of ginger tea or yogi spice tea. Throughout your morning, stay focused and mindful of your energy. Drink two or three glasses of pure water.

Lunch

You are now ready to break your short fast (if you wish to extend it, simply repeat the breakfast routine). Remain mindful of cleansing, however. Have a medium-sized green salad with raw vegetables and two tablespoons of chopped, mixed, raw nuts and five blanched almonds without salt. Use no dressing. Eat slowly, and chew every bite until it dissolves. Introduce food back into your system gently and in small quantities.

Dinner

Have six ounces of freshly squeezed, organic juice half an hour before dinner. A mixture of carrot, celery, and parsley is excellent. Then, enjoy a medium-sized green salad with tomatoes, cucumbers, and a lemon or tomato juice dressing. Don't use oil. For the main course, have three lightly steamed organic vegetables such as string beans, spinach, broccoli, or perhaps some yellow squash with no butter or salt. Use dried herbs such as basil, rosemary, or tarragon for flavoring and to aid digestion. Have another cup of ginger tea or yogi spice tea.

If you get weak or hungry during this short fast, you can do the following.

- Take deep breaths, especially through the left nostril.
- Drink some water.
- Massage your feet with almond oil.
- Do a short meditation. Think about what you're doing, and realize that your feelings of hunger or weakness are temporary. Inhale deeply, hold your breath for five seconds, exhale, and relax.

Chances are, however, that this short fast won't bother you. Rather than feel down, you will feel high and glowing.

If you have the time, you can extend this thirty-six hour fast. I believe, however, that if you want to undertake a prolonged fast or detoxification program, it is best to do so under supervision. The best spots I know for supervised fasts are We Care Holistic Health Ranch in Desert Springs, California, or The Cleanse in Espanola, New Mexico (see page 313 in resource section).

MONODIET AS A FAST

Another way to easily detoxify your system and use food as medicine is to follow a so-called monodiet. In a monodiet, you eat only one food or food combination for a specific purpose for a short time. In the Eat This for That section of this book, I will prescribe a special monodiet or recipe for just about every illness. This should be a key component of your healing program.

BREAKING THE FAST

How you break your fast is critical to the overall success of the fast. It is not unlike coming out of a deep meditation: You must respect your space and especially your stomach and intestines, which have had a nice rest. A double cheese pizza with pepperoni and anchovies is not a good way to make the transition from fasting to eating.

The longer you fast, the clearer you will be mentally, and the more elevated spiritually. Food can bring you down, so take it easy after fasting. A good rule is that for every week you have fasted, you must go slowly and be careful for three days. If you have fasted for only a few days, you must still be cautious for at least forty-eight hours.

When you first break your fast, regardless of its length, avoid potatoes, bananas, white flour, toast, pasta, meats, and cheeses. Also, depending on your constitution, you may want to limit your grain intake to only brown basmati rice. Paradoxically, you may desire all the above foods because your ego is sending a message that it wants you to stop cleansing your body of what you crave. Therefore, stick to watery foods when you first break your fast. Raw or lightly steamed vegetables along with mung beans and brown basmati rice are best.

According to Susana Lombardi, the founder of We Care and the author of *Healthy Living: A Holistic Guide,* the most important part of breaking a fast is to eat small meals. An example is a serving of steamed vegetables, a bowl of soup, and a small salad or piece of fresh fruit. She states that two meals are better than three, and continuing to drink liquids after a fast is vitally important. For that reason, I recommend this formula: Take your body weight, halve the number, and drink that many ounces of fluid daily. For instance, if you weigh 130 pounds, drink 65 ounces of fluid a day, or 2 quarts.

Here is a meal plan to follow a week-long fast. As you will see, it is similar to the meal plan that follows the thirty-six-hour fast.

Breakfast
One glass of organic fruit juice followed 15 minutes later by a piece of organic fruit.

Lunch
One glass of organic vegetable juice followed 15 minutes later by an organic vegetable salad.

Dinner
One cup of yogi tea or herbal tea followed 15 minutes later by a bowl of lightly steamed organic vegetables.

For many patients, I suggest a post-fast monodiet of mung beans and rice. Mung beans are high in natural vegetable protein, rich in important minerals, and very easy to digest. They are an excellent staple that you can use as a healing monodiet or fall back on when you need to regain balance in your life. With the addition of brown basmati rice, steamed vegetables, garlic, onion, ginger, and turmeric, along with a dollop of low-fat yogurt, you have a very nutritious and filling meal. I strongly suggest that you eat it for three days to a week as your main meal after breaking your fast.

Mung Beans and Rice
Makes 8 servings

1 cup mung beans
1 cup basmati rice
2 bay leaves
1-inch piece of kombu seaweed
9 cups of water
4–6 cups chopped assorted vegetables (carrots, celery, zucchini, broccoli, etc.)
2 tablespoons extra virgin olive oil
2 onions, chopped
½ teaspoon pepper
⅓ cup ginger root, minced
3–4 cloves garlic, minced
1 heaping teaspoon turmeric
1 heaping teaspoon garam masala
1 teaspoon crushed red chilies (more or less to taste)

1 tablespoon sweet basil
Seeds of 5 cardamom pods
Sea salt or Braggs Liquid Aminos to taste

Soak beans overnight. Wash beans and rinse rice at least 3 times. Bring water to boil; add beans, bay leaves, and kombu seaweed; and let boil over medium-high flame. When the beans have boiled and are soft, about 40 to 50 minutes, add rice, lower heat to simmer, and let cook for another 20 minutes.

Clean and cut vegetables. Add vegetables to simmering rice and beans and continue to cook for approximately 15 more minutes. In the meantime, heat oil in large frying pan. Add onions, ginger, and garlic, and sauté over medium-high flame until brown. Add turmeric, pepper, garam masala, and red chilies. Add this mixture to the pot with beans and rice. You will need to stir often now to prevent scorching. Add sweet basil, cardamom pods, and sea salt or Braggs to taste. Continue to simmer for another 10 to 15 minutes, stirring often. You may have to add extra boiling water until the rice and vegetables are completely cooked. The consistency should be rich, thick, and souplike, with ingredients barely discernible. Serve with yogurt. This dish is predigested, and is excellent for the sick, the elderly, and young children, but in those cases, make it less spicy. Kombu seaweed enriches this recipe with minerals and helps make the beans more easily digestible.

Simpler Mung Beans and Rice (Kitcheree)
Makes 8 servings

½ cup mung beans
½ cup white basmati rice
1-inch piece of kombu seaweed
9 cups water
Sea salt or Braggs Liquid Aminos to taste

Soak beans overnight. Wash beans and rice. Bring water to boil, add beans and kombu seaweed, and let boil over medium-high flame for approximately 45 to 50 minutes until soft. Then add the rice and let simmer for another 20 to 25 minutes until well done.

Add Braggs or sea salt to taste. You can also add 1 teaspoon of
ghee (recipe found on p. 146) or extra virgin olive oil per person.
Eat with salad and/or steamed vegetables.

TAKE IT EASY

Like anything else in life that's worth doing, detoxifying your system may
take a bit of time, practice, and effort. But that's all right. The process and
the journey are as important as the final destination. As you cleanse your
system, please do not stress over it. Move slowly away from alarm foods and
toward health-promoting and calming foods. Because low-stress foods—
lots of steamed, organic vegetables—are easy to prepare, they don't require
a lot of time or great sophistication in the kitchen. You are limited only by
your imagination, which is boundless, and your desire and motivation to be
healthy, strong, relaxed, and happy.

Remember how great you feel at the end of the fast. Try to keep that
feeling by allowing for one holy day a week, similar to a Sabbath, when you
return to the fasting state. Perhaps this day can be your Sabbath—therefore, why not fast on Saturday or Sunday, depending on your religion? As a
Sikh, I look forward to our Sunday service to be with the community, but
because of the delicious vegetarian meal that is part of this event it would
be impractical for me to fast on that day. So I usually fast on Wednesdays.
It works for me. Please decide what works for you, and try it.

CHAPTER 9

The Second Principle: Go Organic

Once you break your cleansing fast and begin a new diet that's rich in phytonutrient-dense fresh fruits and vegetables, it's important that you go organic. The main reason for doing so is to ensure that you are getting pure food, untainted by pesticides. There is no role in a healthy, life-affirming regimen for substances designed to poison and kill. It's that simple.

Pesticides may be a contributing factor to a long list of serious diseases, including Parkinson's, leukemia, non-Hodgkin's lymphoma, and cancers of the brain, stomach, and prostate gland. Medical research has also revealed a correlation between the increase in the use of pesticides and the rise in breast cancer among American women, almost certainly because pesticides have an abnormal estrogenic effect that leads to cancer. According to the Environmental Protection Agency's own research, more than 107 different active ingredients in pesticides are known or probable carcinogens. Approximately 2.2 billion pounds of pesticides are used in America every year—about 8 pounds for every man, woman, and child.

Serving organic rather than conventional foods may be most beneficial to your children. Many childhood favorites such as peanut butter, peaches, grapes, raisins, apples, milk, and cereal are among the foods most heavily treated with chemicals. This is hazardous to the developing immune and nervous systems of small children and can make them extremely susceptible to pesticide toxicity. Exposure to these substances during a critical stage of development can permanently weaken or change the function of any of a child's organ systems. This may be what's behind the 300 percent increase in childhood brain cancer and leukemia during the past twenty-five years, as the number and concentration of pesticides have risen. Cancer now kills more children under age 14 than any other disease. Biting into a single nonorganic apple can expose a child to the residues of thirty-four different pesticides.

The tragedy is that the Environmental Protection Agency essentially ignores childhood exposure to combinations of pesticides, including those in contaminated water. Our government's policy is based on the idea that a certain number of deaths from pesticides and such is *acceptable* in order to protect the interests of big business and the conventional food industry. An additional chilling fact is that according to published reports, 95 percent of mother's milk has become tainted with pesticides.

The good news is that using primarily organic food can reverse all this. What do the terms *organically grown* or *certified organic* actually mean? They mean that the bright red strawberry you are about to eat would not contain 70 different pesticides, since strawberries are the most heavily sprayed crop. The second most heavily sprayed crop is coffee; DDT, malathion, and other deadly pesticides are part of your wake-up brew unless you drink organic. Tobacco is another heavily sprayed crop, so pesticides can be added to the list of poisons a smoker is inhaling with each puff.

To be certified as organic, a farmer's land must be chemical-free for at least three years. In October 2002 the USDA replaced state or private certification with national standards, which confirm that the farmer is following the organic philosophy both in methods and in materials. This program has set national standards for certification, awarded only when no artificial substances go into the food as it is grown or processed. No pesticides can be sprayed on grapes, for example, even as they leave the farm en route to market. Beyond that, under the national organic legislation of 1996, a grocery item such as soup or frozen dinner can be labeled organic only if it contains a minimum of 95 percent of organic ingredients. When organic ingredients make up at least 50 percent of the product, a company can list them on the front label; anything less can be listed only on the side panel. This certification program has proved to be very successful, and less than .01 percent of certified organic farms ever have their certifications revoked. To make sure the food you buy is organic, look for the words "certified organic." The use of other slogans such as *natural, pesticide-free,* or anything else does not mean the food is organic.

From a health standpoint, organically grown food is higher in minerals than conventional food. For example, organic food contains many times more calcium, chromium, magnesium, and selenium than food grown with pesticides. There have been reports of illnesses such as allergies, asthma, eczema, and chemical sensitivities, among others, totally reversing when the patient switched to organic foods.

Organic food tastes better than food treated with pesticides and, contrary to one popular myth, is not more expensive in many parts of the United States, such as the northwest and southwest. A landmark 1995 study conducted by the organization Mothers and Others for a Livable Planet showed that depending upon where you live, organic food may cost the same or less than conventionally grown produce. Depending upon where you live, organic foods may be even more reasonably priced if you buy them in bulk from a farmer's market or food co-op. In my view, even if organic food does cost more, the benefits to your health and that of the environment make it well worthwhile.

BEYOND YOUR OWN HEALTH BENEFITS: GOING ORGANIC FOR THE HEALTH OF PLANET EARTH

That's right—there's more to going organic than your own health and that of your family. A switch to organic food is vital if we're to save our environment. Organically farmed soil is alive, not depleted of its mineral content and other natural substances. Healthy soil creates strong, vibrant plants that help produce healthy people. Conventional farmers treat their soil as nothing more than an anchor for root plants, and the land gradually becomes hard, dry, unproductive, and vulnerable to rapid erosion. Conventional farming practices destroy three billion tons of topsoil every year—a rate seven times faster than Mother Nature can replenish.

The organic farmer has a different, earth-friendly philosophy. Organic farmers feed their soil with compost and manure, in the manner of nature itself. This approach allows the plants to become more resistant to pests and disease. Organic farmers work in harmony with nature to keep insect populations in check. They use birds and ladybugs, which feast on annoying pests, and they plant flower borders to fool other insects. All of this means better food, healthier bodies, and clearer minds.

Organic farming is increasing worldwide at a faster pace than it is here at home. Currently in the United States, although organic acreage is increasing rapidly, only 0.2 percent of the nation's crops are grown on organic land. Compare that with the European Union, where, according to the Worldwatch Institute, organic farming will account for 30 percent of the total farmed area by 2010. Slowly, going organic is being recognized as an important component of a healthy lifestyle.

You can even extend the concept of going organic to the animal products you buy. Recent investigations have shown that conventionally raised beef, for example, is loaded with hormones, antibiotics, and pesticides. Cattle raised in a manner called free range, as we'll see in chapter 11, tastes better and is better for your health.

CHAPTER 10

The Third Principle: Limit or Eliminate Genetically Engineered Foods

The commercial cultivation of genetically engineered (GE) foods, also called genetically modified organisms (GMO), has become big business. Such crops offer the potential benefits of higher yields and lower chemical pesticide usage, but they may also harm agriculture, the environment, and human health, according to many well-researched articles in respected journals such as *Nature* and *Environment*.

WHAT ARE GENETICALLY ENGINEERED FOODS?

Creating genetically engineered foods involves permanently changing the blueprint of a living organism by manipulating its DNA. In this process, an alien gene is inserted into a plant to give it potentially useful new traits, such as tolerance for herbicides or the ability to kill insects that feed on it. Besides plants, this can be done with vegetables, fruits, seeds, animals, and, perhaps someday, human beings. Research scientists and business people, principally from very large multinational companies such as Monsanto, one of the largest and most profitable agribusinesses, and Dow Chemical, among others, do this work. A company will modify and then patent the genes of a seed, for example, then sell the seeds and gain control of a market share.

Genetically engineered food is a potential problem because genetic material can now be transferred between species that would never interbreed in nature. Moreover, GMO technology is still unpredictable and imprecise. Because of that, it may turn out to be dangerous to your health. For example, a common genetically engineered corn was designed to carry a toxic pesticide to ward off an insect called a corn borer. The potential danger comes when you drink the milk or eat the meat from a cow that eats this corn. In that case you may absorb this pesticide with all its inherent possible dangers of altered immunity, allergies, and perhaps even cancer.

ARE GENETICALLY ENGINEERED FOODS SAFE TO EAT?

That is a key question, especially since 70 percent of the food on grocery store shelves across America is already genetically engineered. Unfortunately, no long-term studies of GE foods have been conducted on humans, and the United States government hasn't required testing. Most of the available evidence, however, is leading scientists and environmental organizations to caution us about eating GE foods. At present, it is almost unknown how the technologies that create GE foods—such as recombinant DNA, in which plant genes are inserted into unrelated species—will affect us.

Because no long-term studies on humans have been done, the British Medical Association and many independent scientists have called for a moratorium on the sale and consumption of GE foods until further research is undertaken. Exploring the research that exists, however, leads us to a body of evidence indicating that GE foods may cause toxic exposure to allergens and also elevate our risk of cancer.

A major independent feeding study on rats, done by Arpud Pusztai, Ph.D., at the renowned Rowett Institute in Scotland, revealed very serious adverse effects of GE foods. Dr. Pusztai had been a proponent of GE foods before doing his research, but what he found was very shocking to the British public, who read about the study in page one stories throughout late 1998 and early 1999.

Dr. Pusztai's research discovered that genetically engineered potatoes had poisoned laboratory rats. After ten days, the GE potatoes damaged the rodents' vital organs and immune systems, while the rats that ate normal potatoes were unharmed. The conclusion was that something, as yet unidentified, in the GE procedure turned the potatoes into a virulent poison. The scientists theorized that the damage to the rats' intestines and stomach linings most likely had been caused by a severe viral infection produced by the standard chemical switch used in all GE food and crops.

You would expect Dr. Pusztai's groundbreaking research to have been rewarded, but the opposite occurred. His work remains incomplete to this day because his funding was cut off in October 1999, after his studies were published in *Lancet,* one of the world's leading medical journals. An article published shortly thereafter in the *Guardian,* a leading British newspaper, implied that Pusztai's research had threatened the powerful biotech scientific establishment.

Since then, many internationally recognized scientists have sided with Dr. Pusztai. They have warned that many of the common GE foods that you and your family eat daily may be hazardous to your health. On May 17, 1999, the 115,000-member British Medical Association issued a report calling for a halt to the production of genetically engineered foods and crops. The report stated that more research was needed to assess the safety of GE foods and warned that the sale of untested GE foods could lead to the development of new allergies and antibiotic resistance in humans.

Later that same year, as documented in the book *Genetically Engineered Foods* by Ronnie Cummins and Ben Lilliston, 231 scientists from 31 countries published an open letter to all governments calling for a halt to genetic engineering. The scientists emphasized that the virus used to change the genetic makeup of the food could potentially generate new viruses that cause disease. As testing on GE foods is still incomplete, it is unknown to this day whether they are safe to eat.

ARE GENETICALLY ENGINEERED FOODS SAFE FOR THE ENVIRONMENT?

At this moment, millions of acres of genetically engineered crops are under cultivation in the United States, and untold damage is already being done to the land. Not unlike the effects of GE foods on human health, the long-term result of genetic engineering on the earth's ecosystem is unclear. Evidence that GE foods are harming the environment is, however, rapidly accumulating.

The worst problem is that the effect of GE food on the environment is irreversible. Genetic pollution, unlike air and water pollution, cannot simply be cleaned up, because crops are living organisms. Once genetically engineered plants have been introduced, they spread their altered genetic material to other plants. Because they are alive, moreover, they can also reproduce and mutate. This genetic drift is already polluting the DNA of organic and non–genetically engineered plants, according to several published research studies. For example, in a 1994 issue of the journal *Science*, James Kling documented the spread of herbicide-resistant canola plant genes into mustard plants in a distant field. A 1999 study by the Soil Association of the United Kingdom found pollen of genetically engineered rapeseed plants more than three miles away from the original plant. According to the authors, bees had transported it there.

In May 1999, in one of the most renowned articles about genetic engineering ever published in *Nature* magazine, Cornell University scientists stated that when monarch butterflies ate milkweed leaves, their sole food source, that had been dusted with pollen from GE corn, 44 percent died. The survivors suffered a 60 percent weight loss. To the authors of this project, this underscored the need for more research on genetically engineered crops.

Monsanto immediately tried to discredit this work, complaining that the studies were carried out in a laboratory rather than in the field. Further study by scientists from Iowa State University conducted on monarch butterflies in the field, however, showed a 19 percent mortality rate within 48 hours after the butterflies ate the polluted milkweed. Other studies have shown that beneficial insects such as ladybugs, as well as insect-eating birds, are also being killed. Beyond that, genetically engineered crops appear to damage soil fertility by killing microorganisms.

In sum, the long-term effects of genetically engineered crops on the soil, insects, and animal life are not yet completely understood, but they are not without signs of danger.

SHOULD GENETICALLY ENGINEERED FOODS BE LABELED?

Genetically engineered seeds use up to five times more herbicide than non-GE seeds, according to one study of more than eight thousand university-based field trials. Moreover, scientists at an international meeting in Switzerland in March 1999 pointed out that some GE crops exude ten to twenty times the amount of toxins contained in conventional crops. The scientists at that meeting called for a moratorium on commercial planting of GE crops that use these toxic chemicals. As of this date, however, there has been no reduction; in fact, an increase has occurred in the production of GE crops and foods in this country.

That's only one part of the problem. The critical issue is that we have no way of knowing whether the food we buy and eat has been genetically modified or not, because the United States government does not require it to be labeled. Somehow, the large biotech companies have convinced our politicians and regulatory agencies that GE foods are no different from conventional foods. And, their logic goes, since conventional foods don't have to be labeled, then neither should GE foods require labeling. This is a very serious issue, one that has many scientists and environmental organizations such as Greenpeace and Mothers for Natural Law doing whatever they can to educate the public. Support for labeling also comes from conventional physician writers such as Michael Roizen, M.D., and John La Palma, M.D. (also a master chef), authors of the book *The Real Age Diet,* who call for labeling of GE foods. Integrative medicine guru Andrew Weil, M.D., author of numerous books on health, food, and healing, also supports labeling of GE foods.

I believe we have the right to know whether the food we eat is genetically engineered. This right has already been extended to the people of Japan and the European Union, where GE labeling is almost universally required.

Here's a look at what our government is allowing biotechnology companies to unleash upon an unsuspecting public:

- Potatoes that glow when they need to be watered, thanks to jellyfish genes that have been added
- GMO-enhanced salmon that are twice as large as any known to science
- Vegetables with scorpion genes
- Pigs with human genes
- Tomatoes with flounder genes
- GMO cows that produce human breast milk

WHICH PRODUCTS AND FOODS CONTAIN GMOS?

The only way you can be certain you're not eating GE foods is to follow the second principle and go organic. To do that, you will need to look for food that is labeled non-GMO. If you eat lots of organic fruits and vegetables, you will be well on your way to guaranteed healthy nutrition. Even if you eat meat, chicken, and fish, there are ways to avoid animals that have been raised on genetically engineered (GE or GMO) feed. To be an informed shopper, read labels and be diligent.

One fast way to begin eliminating GMO from your diet is to avoid all processed foods, particularly those containing corn, canola, and soy (this doesn't include non-GMO tofu or soy burgers).

Research by the Organic Consumers Association suggests that at least 60 percent of processed foods contains ingredients derived from genetically engineered soybeans alone. Because of space limitations, I can't possibly list all the GE foods and derivatives out there, but I can name enough to help you. You can then log onto my website, www.drdharma.com, to learn more.

The following list of GMO foods is based on the work of the nonprofit organization Mothers for Natural Law. It will increase your awareness of the GE problem and highlight its ubiquitousness.

- **Aspartame (also known as NutraSweet)**—This is a GMO chemical, usually found in diet soft drinks, that is also in over nine thousand other products, including children's vitamins and medicines, chewing gum, and many low-fat products such as jelly, jam, and yogurt. It is also found in some candy.

- **Canola**—Besides canola oil itself, canola derivatives may be found in chips, salad dressings, cookies, margarine, soy cheeses, and fried foods.

- **Corn**—Derivatives of corn include corn syrup, corn fructose, cornstarch, corn dextrose, corn oil, and corn flour. Products that may contain genetically engineered corn derivatives include vitamin C, tofu dogs, tortilla chips, candy, ice cream, infant formula, salad dressing, tomato sauce, bread, cookies, cereals, baking powder, alcohol, vanilla, margarine, soy sauce, tamari, soda, fried foods, powdered sugar, enriched flour, and pasta. Other products derived from

GMO corn include dextrose, glucose, maltose, sucrose, and sugars used in canned fruit and soft drinks. Maltodextrin, an industrial carbohydrate filler derived from corn, is found in fillers such as gravy mixes and flavored chips as well as cooked processed meats such as sliced ham and chicken, and in dry baby foods. Xanthan gum (E415) comes from corn sugar and is used as a thickener in ice cream, salad dressings, and confectionery.

- **Cotton**—Cottonseed oil may be found in vegetable oil as well as in products such as chips, peanut butter, crackers, and cookies.

- **Crook-necked yellow squash**—This vegetable, which can be found in whole form or in baby food, may be GMO.

- **Dairy products**—Milk, cheese, butter, buttermilk, sour cream, yogurt, and whey are all currently GMO unless you buy organic. Also, milk from cows injected with the recombinant bovine growth hormone (rBGH) is often mixed together with conventionally produced milk, creating an identification problem.

- **Papaya**—Currently the only GMO fruit. Others in development include apples, grapes, strawberries (the food most heavily laden with pesticides), pineapples, bananas, and melons.

- **Potatoes**—The russet Burbank is the only GMO variety at the moment. There are products, however, that contain GMO potatoes such as french fries, mashed potatoes, chips, and potato mixes. Some potato Passover products, potato-vegetable pies, and potato soups also contain GMO derivatives.

- **Soybeans**—Derivatives include lecithin, soybean oil, soy flour, soy protein, soy isolates, and genistein. Lecithin E322 is the most common additive in food. It is used in bread and baked goods, chocolate, margarine, cheese spread, mayonnaise, powdered milk, baby formula, cream, cheese spreads, fresh pasta, and more. Tofu dogs, cereals, veggie burgers, and many other products also contain GMO soy isolates. Therefore, always look for products labeled non-GMO. For example, just this morning I had a protein smoothie in which I used a non-GMO protein powder from Whole Foods Market.

- **Tomatoes**—Both regular and cherry tomatoes may be GMO. Products that may contain GMO tomatoes or derivatives are tomato sauces and purees, pizza, lasagna, and processed Italian and Mexican foods.

On www.drdharma.com, I list many other foods testing positive for GMO. I also name the food companies using GMO and those that don't.

Remember—your first line of defense against the dangers of genetically engineered foods is to go organic.

Now is the time to become proactive in stopping GMO. I ask you to support the anti-GMO organizations I have listed in the resource section of this book and on my website. It is the only way we can hold back the powerful biotechnology companies from forcing any more GE foods onto our plate.

FOOD LOG EXERCISE #9

At an airport restaurant I ordered a salad with Italian dressing, which came in a plastic pouch. Now that you've read about the importance of organic foods and the prevalence of genetically engineered foods, what do you think of these ingredients?

Soybean oil (GMO), water, red wine vinegar (preserved with sulfites), sugar, salt, Parmesan cheese (contains growth hormones and pesticides), enzymes, calcium chloride, red bell peppers (pesticides), onion (pesticides), xanthan gum, beet juice (pesticides), garlic, celery seed (GMO), propylene glycol, alginate, and calcium disodium EDTA added to protect flavor.

This concoction has 150 calories, of which 140 are from fat. It also has 500 mg of sodium. Would you eat it?

CHAPTER II

The Fourth Principle: Eat Clean Protein

My good friend Nordine Zouareg of Paris is a two-time Mr. Universe body-building champion. Nordine eats a high-protein diet because of his intense training schedule. His diet, however, is low in fat. At first glance you might say, "Impossible," but you'd be wrong. Not only is a high-protein, low-fat diet realistic, but in my clinical experience it's also crucial if your goal is maximum health.

Personally and professionally, I believe in a high-protein diet as part of a lifestyle program that includes adequate exercise. (A lower-protein diet is advisable if you don't exercise.) Some doctors say that eating a diet high in protein can cause liver or kidney damage, but I've never seen or heard about an actual, as opposed to hypothetical, case. Of course, if someone already has such an ailment, I wouldn't suggest a high-protein diet.

Many times in my clinical practice, however, I have seen people complaining of low energy, fatigue, depression, anxiety, poor memory, and moodiness when they do not eat enough protein. For this reason, I have my nutritionist work with my patients to construct a diet containing around 40 percent protein, depending on activity level. The diet also contains 15 to 20 percent fat, rich in the salubrious omega-3 fats from both vegetarian sources, such as flaxseeds, and non-vegetarian sources, such as salmon and other oily fish. The remainder of the plan consists of complex carbohydrates such as grains, nuts, seeds, and organic fruits and vegetables. This dietary program is also naturally low in calories, which as you will recall is itself life extending.

What is unique about my program is that I help you move away from eating too much animal protein, as found in conventionally raised red meat, and toward lean free-range meat or chicken, fish, non-GMO soy (including tofu), and protein supplements. It is important to point out that my studies, clinical experience, and scientific research have revealed that the closer one eats to a vegetarian diet the better his or her health. I realize, however, that many of you may not be ready to become vegetarians or may not even want to do so. I want you to stick with your healthy diet—and, just as important, enjoy it. When you are happy with what you are eating, it becomes not a diet but a way of life. Therefore, when a healing partner is reluctant to move toward vegetarianism or wants to make it a slow transition, I tell that person about the importance of clean protein and a natural approach to meat, poultry, and seafood.

To understand the concept of clean protein, recall the rules of certification for organic foods, which state that it is free from pesticides. According to the Environmental Protection Agency, 90 to 95 percent of all pesticide residues are found in meat, fish, and dairy products. Therefore, it is of vital importance to educate yourself to recognize pesticide-free meat.

The word used to signify organic meat is *natural,* but you must be cautious, especially in a traditional supermarket. In a conventional sense, *natural* applies only to processing and means that the product contains no artificial preservatives. It tells you nothing about the use of pesticides, antibiotics, or growth hormones. However, at modern health food supermarkets such as Wild Oats, Whole Foods, Trader Joe's, and others, the word *natural* has come to signify that the animals have been raised and processed in a healthy way.

The animals are humanely raised. The animals have ample room to move about in a paddock or are free range, meaning that they are unconfined and graze on local vegetation. When animals are raised in stress-free living conditions, they are leaner, containing approximately 20 percent less fat. Free-range meat is also better tasting and more tender. Crowded feedlots are sprayed heavily with pesticides to control flies. These pesticides end up in the meat you eat and then in your body, where their unhealthy effects may not be apparent for years.

The animals are raised drug-free. Conventional meat producers use a wide variety of FDA-approved drugs, as well as an unknown number of other dangerous substances for which a prescription from a veterinarian is not needed.

The meat is antibiotic-free. Animals raised in conventional feedlots automatically receive antibiotics to counteract the unclean conditions on factory farms. As a result, many strains of bacteria including *E. coli* and *Salmonella* are becoming increasingly resistant to all available antibiotics. Three studies published in the *New England Journal Of Medicine* in late 2001 confirmed that the routine use of antibiotics to enhance growth in farm animals may encourage the growth of drug-resistant bacteria. The Union of Concerned Scientists, a nonprofit group based in Cambridge, Massachusetts, estimated that 26.6 million pounds of antibiotics are administered to animals each year, while only 2 million pounds are needed to treat active infections. The rest of the antibiotics are used needlessly to prevent infection or promote growth. Although the FDA has for years tried to tighten controls over the use of antibiotics on farm animals, a practice the European Union banned in 1998, they are meeting organized opposition from meat industry executives. As an example, Ron Phillips, a spokesman for the Animal Health Institute, a trade group representing manufacturers of veterinary drugs, was quoted as saying, "The way to manage antibiotic resistance is not by banning products but by judicious use and robust surveillance which gives an information base on which to make informed management decisions. Antibiotics are used to raise healthy animals. They're vitally important to deliver a safe, wholesome supply of meat to the American consumer."

Meanwhile, a study by scientists at the University of Maryland and the FDA in 2001 examined 200 samples of ground meats—chicken, beef, turkey, and pork—from three conventional supermarkets in the Washington, D.C., area. *Salmonella,* a leading cause of food poisoning, contaminated a fifth of the samples. Antibiotic resistance was rampant among the contaminated samples, with 84 percent resistant to at least one antibiotic and 53 percent resistant to at least three. One microorganism, an especially virulent strain of *Salmonella,* had become a "superbug," resistant to twelve antibiotics.

In the paper describing this study, its director, Dr. J. Meng of the University of Miami, stated the obvious: "The agricultural sector is not doing a very good job of controlling the emergence of resistant organisms."

No artificial growth hormones are used. Conventional meat processors love to give their cows growth hormones. It is a great investment. These drugs produce monster animals, larger than nature ever intended.

Unfortunately for the consumer, the consumption of meat raised using these drugs can lead to bizarre effects in people, including the onset of precocious puberty in five-year-old girls and the development of cancer years later.

The animals are raised on a natural grassy diet. Cows are innately vegetarian. Diseases such as mad cow disease are caused by animal feed containing diseased parts of fellow beasts.

The animals have a low-stress environment. Animals raised under typical conditions on large factory farms are stressed out. They are constantly in an alarm state. This causes them to release stress hormones such as adrenaline in large amounts. Adrenaline and other stress hormones released in response to fear of impending doom causes the animals' tissues to harden and turn dark. Their meat is tougher and less appetizing than that from humanely raised creatures.

NONTRADITIONAL MEAT SOURCES

The meats with the least fat come from more exotic sources such as buffalo, rabbit, ostrich, and venison. These sources of clean protein have fewer calories and cholesterol than other red meats and no residues of antibiotics or growth hormones. The downside of eating some of these more exotic types of animal protein is that they are more expensive and difficult to find. However, turkey is much more reasonably priced and may be found in the natural and antibiotic-free state. It is low in fat and contains tryptophan, the essential amino acid that regulates metabolism and induces sleep.

MEAT HANDLING GUIDELINES

- Never eat raw meat.
- After handling meat, wash your hands, utensils, cutting board, and any other surface thoroughly with hot soapy water.
- Keep raw meat and anything it touches away from ready-to-eat foods.

- Defrost meat in the refrigerator. If you defrost it using a microwave, cook the thawed meat immediately.
- Storage times for raw poultry are no more than two or three days in the coldest part of the refrigerator; for raw ground beef, two or three days; for fresh fish, one or two days.
- Always cook meat to an internal temperature of 160°F. This applies especially to poultry and ground meats, which carry surface bacteria.
- Refrigerate leftover meat immediately in small containers that cool quickly. Use or freeze the meat within three days.

CHICKEN HANDLING GUIDELINES

- Always follow the safe-handling guidelines for meat.
- Never eat pink chicken; make sure it is cooked all the way through.
- Avoid deep-frying and pan-frying chicken.

MEAT PRODUCTS IN UNEXPECTED PLACES

As with GMO products, meat may end up in places you'd never expect it. We realized that the french fries at McDonald's contained beef extract only when Eric Schlosser documented it in his book *Fast Food Nation.* An article in *Business Week* also disclosed that many other seemingly meat-free foods contain animal products. Surprisingly, Kellogg's Frosted Mini-Wheats contain meat in the form of gelatin. Gelatin, as you recall, is a gummy substance rendered from cattle carcasses. It's also used to coat pills. For example, I remember having to confirm that a product I designed for a vitamin company was vegetarian and therefore free of gelatin. Gelatin can also be found in marshmallows, sour cream, Skittles, and other candies as well as in Jell-O.

Many restaurants also include animal ingredients without your knowledge. As of this writing, Church's Chicken and Denny's flavor their fries with meat fat. The guacamole at Applebee's contains gelatin, and its vegetable roll-up tortillas contain lard, which is pork fat. Pizza Hut only recently eliminated chicken broth from its pizza sauce but still uses it in its white sauce in pasta dishes.

As you recall, many of these ingredients may be GMO, which delivers a double blow: You are eating food with unknown potential side effects that also contains higher than expected amounts of animal fat. For someone interested in moving toward a mostly (or totally) vegetarian lifestyle, this is disturbing and highlights the need to know what you are eating before you bite.

FISH

Fish is becoming ever more popular as a source of healthy protein. It is high in protein but low in saturated fat, and it is an excellent source of selenium, zinc, iodine, essential fatty acids, niacin, and vitamins B_6 and B_{12}. As you may know, recent studies have shown that the fat contained in fish—omega-3 fatty acids, as they are known—is very good for you. Omega-3s increase good cholesterol and decrease bad cholesterol, and some researchers suggest that this fat also reduces triglyceride levels. This is crucial to maximum health because low triglycerides decrease the risk of hardening of the arteries (atherosclerosis) and thereby reduce your chance of having a heart attack. Eating fish once a week or more often provides a 44 percent lower risk of having a fatal heart attack, according to David Siscovick, M.D., a professor at the University of Washington School of Medicine in Seattle.

There are several theories about why omega-3s are so heart healthy. Mine is that they make your blood platelets less sticky, making it harder for blood clots to attach to the walls of arteries of your heart and brain. Omega-3 fats also help maintain your heart's normal rhythm—an important benefit because irregular heart function may lead to sudden death by cardiac collapse or stroke.

Omega-3 fats from fish may also reduce the risk of breast and colon cancer. Moreover, fish oils help reduce inflammation, thus improving the functional mobility of patients with rheumatoid arthritis and similar painful conditions. Eating fish regularly has also proved helpful in eliminating the agonizing symptoms of Crohn's disease, an inflammatory condition of the bowel. Saturated fat sends a signal of inflammation to your body, whereas omega-3 fats block that very signal.

A great deal of research suggests that all healthy diets should include omega-3 fatty acids from fish or vegetarian sources. Omega-3s are very good for your mental function. My colleague William Grant, Ph.D., is a brilliant scientist who works for NASA. When his mother was diagnosed with Alzheimer's disease, he undertook a computerized review of the World Health Organization literature. He discovered that diets high in saturated fat, such as those found in red meat, lead to a higher risk of Alzheimer's. He also discovered that in countries where there is a high consumption of omega-3 fats, the rates of this dreaded disease are markedly reduced.

In addition, scientists think they have evidence that omega-3s can cure mental disorders such as depression and dyslexia. Alexandra Richardson, M.D., Senior Neuroscience Fellow at Britain's Oxford University, put it simply at a seminar for fellow physicians when she said, "If the brain does not have the right fats, it will not work well." Richardson's research found that the lack of omega-3 fatty acids may directly correlate to the development of depression, autism, dyslexia, and attention deficit hyperactivity disorder (ADHD) in some people.

I find a fascinating correlation between Dr. Richardson's work concerning depression and Dr. Grant's research concerning memory loss. It confirms my own experience in treating patients with these disorders, using supplements of DHA, an omega-3 oil derived from algae.

If you choose to make fish a significant protein source in your diet, there are important points to remember. Fried fish of any kind is not part of a healthy diet. For one thing, fried cod, catfish, and snapper do not contain significant omega-3 fat. Beyond that, fried foods send a pro-inflammatory message to your genes, leading to a predisposition to mutation, which may lead to cancer.

WHAT ABOUT FARMED FISH?

The debate rages over whether farmed fish is safer, healthier, or better tasting than fish caught in the wild. I explored this question by visiting a Wild Oats market in Tucson. I looked at the wild salmon and then looked at the farmed variety. It was obvious that the salmon from the wilds of the northern Pacific Ocean off the coast of Alaska had deeper-colored and richer-looking meat than its farmed counterpart. The wild salmon meat was deep red; the meat of the farmed fish was light pink. Wild salmon apparently tastes better, too. I'm sure it's because farmed fish are penned like conventionally raised meat and chicken. They are inoculated against disease and fed on pellets of soy meal (GMO), corn gluten (GMO), and oil (GMO).

And what about that nice pink color? Their feed contains an artificial pigment.

Millions of farmed salmon, in a manner similar to some GMO seeds that contaminate non-GMO seeds, have escaped from farms over the years and have appeared in rivers in British Columbia and southern Alaska, where they have contaminated native species. Farmed salmon are also said to carry disease despite being dosed with antibiotics. The scariest part is that some farm companies are experimenting with genetic engineering to speed the growth of the fish.

Be cautious when selecting the fish you eat. In 2002, the world production of farmed salmon is estimated to exceed 1.2 million metric tons, up from about 250,000 tons in 1990. Wild salmon equals only about 750,000 metric tons.

DANGERS OF WILD FISH

Some wild fish, most notably shark, swordfish, and tuna, also have potential problems with contamination. They may contain mercury, lead, cadmium, chromium, and arsenic. My major concern is for our children. Toxins from fish may be stored in a woman's body for longer than six years and then passed to her children through the placenta or breast milk.

My suggestion is to be selective. Go for the wild salmon or other oily fish because of their high protein content and richness in omega-3s, and buy it in a health food supermarket if possible.

Many exotic types of fish found in seafood restaurants are flown in daily from Hawaii. They are very tasty and are probably quite safe. But for the most part, when you go food shopping, you are going to have to consider the facts: Both farm-raised and wild fish may be dangerous to your long-term health.

SOME FINAL SUGGESTIONS ON EATING FISH

- Eat a variety of fish to lessen your risk of overdosing on one contaminated source.
- Eat fish only two or three times a week.
- Remove the skin, a major source of toxins.
- Preferably choose wild ocean fish harvested far from shore.
- Select fresh salmon caught during the Alaskan salmon season (May through September).

- During the off season, choose frozen Alaskan salmon, which is usually cleaned and frozen immediately after being caught.
- If you eat trout or catfish, go with the farmed versions because the wild fish are caught in streams, rivers, and lakes that tend to be more polluted.
- Choose smaller fish because they are less toxic.
- If you're pregnant, don't eat more than 7 ounces of canned tuna a week, and don't eat swordfish, shark, fresh tuna, or fish from inland waters more than once a month.

Food	Portion Size	Protein Grams	Fat Grams
Red meat	3 oz.	23	13
Chicken (broiled)	½ breast	26	3
Pork	3 oz.	22	14
Salmon	3 oz.	23	9
Tuna (in water)	3 oz.	21	0.7
Turkey	3 oz.	25	2
Hamburger	3 oz.	20	17
Tofu (firm)	½ block	12	6 (not bad fat)
Nuts (almonds)	1 oz.	6	14
Beans	1 cup	15	0.8
Rice	1 cup	4	0.4

USDA Nutrient Database for Standard Reference, Release 14, 2001.

SOY PROTEIN

As you can see from the preceding chart, soy is a very healthful, safe, high-protein alternative to animal protein. It is found in several forms, including white block tofu, precooked tofu burgers, soybean pods (edamame), and soy turkey, ham, pepperoni, and even Canadian bacon. It can also be found in soymilk, soy cereal, and soy nuts. I especially love making a daily breakfast smoothie with soy protein powder.

Soy is an excellent dietary choice because it contains a high amount of protein and is low in saturated fat and cholesterol. Just 25 mg of soy a day protects against heart disease. In 1995, the *New England Journal of Medicine* reported that consuming 47 grams of soy protein a day (about 2 ounces) reduced blood cholesterol by 10 percent in one month. In subjects with very elevated cholesterol levels, above 300, it was lowered as much as 20 percent. Those 2 ounces of soy also protect against prostate cancer, breast cancer, lung cancer, colon cancer, and menopausal problems.

A study published in the May 2001 issue of *Cancer, Epidemiology, Biomarkers, and Prevention* looked at the relationship between soy intake during adolescence and the risk of breast cancer later in life. For each incremental increase in soy intake during adolescence in females, there was a reduction in the risk of breast cancer. Women with the highest consumption of soy had only half the risk of those with the lowest intake. There is one word of caution, however. While soy does protect against breast cancer development, there is some concern among researchers, based primarily on animal and laboratory research, that soy may stimulate breast tumors once they occur. I suggest therefore, that women with breast cancer not eat soy products.

It is easy to gradually work soy into your diet by replacing one daily serving of animal protein with tofu. Also remember that if you shop at a health food store, you can easily find non-GMO soy. For example, Mori-Nu block tofu is an especially good product because it is made with certified organic non-GMO soybeans. Being organic and non-GMO means that no preservatives are used in its manufacturing process, and it is not irradiated. Mori-Nu also contains the full spectrum of naturally occurring soy isoflavones, including genestein, phytic acids, saponins, and protease inhibitors, all of which are key constituents in making soy healthful.

Besides being high in protein and low in fat, soy products contain a good amount of calcium, which is so important for keeping bones healthy with age, especially in women. Food scientists have also found many antioxidant compounds in soy foods that protect against free radical damage. Other important compounds found in soy include vitamin E, phosphorus, and coenzyme Q10, which plays a very important role in cellular energy dynamics. Even iron is found in tofu.

By substituting soy for red meat, you are improving your health because soybeans are equivalent to animal foods in protein quality and quantity, but without the saturated fat.

SOURCES OF SOY PROTEIN

There are many interesting ways to reap the benefits of soy in addition to preparing it from white blocks of tofu or eating it in the form of a meat substitute.

Tempeh

Tempeh is a traditional Indonesian food that has meatlike texture and a deep, rich flavor. Tempeh is made from soybeans that are first cultured and fermented, and then pressed into cakes. I recall many years ago beginning a strenuous weight-lifting program and craving meat. Having become a vegetarian seven years previously, I asked Yogi Bhajan what to do. He suggested that I drink 16 ounces of cucumber juice daily to balance the minerals in my brain and eat tempeh with nine-grain bread. I complied with his instructions, and the cravings for meat subsided. In fact, I felt great and had enough energy to continue with my weight-training program.

Tempeh provides the highest-quality plant source of protein. It is easily digested and assimilated into your body, sending wonderful, healthy signals to your cells and genes. Tempeh is loaded with protein, containing 17 grams per 4-ounce serving. It is rich in fiber, B vitamins, calcium, and iron. If you are looking for increased strength and athletic endurance, my advice is to eat more tempeh.

There is only one rule to follow when you eat tempeh. Cook it before you eat it. That may sound strange, but some people, including my daughter Hari, like to eat block tofu raw. That is not recommended in yoga nutritional therapy because both raw tofu and raw tempeh are indigestible.

Miso

Have you ever had miso soup at a Japanese restaurant? If so, you are aware of its wonderful flavor, aroma, and heartiness. Miso is a fermented soybean paste made from cooked soybeans, salt, water, and a special grain called koji. When I eat miso soup I can feel it bringing its nutritional goodness to my cells. One cup can reduce harmful blood acidity and prevent the cellular damage that occurs daily from pollution and radiation. Because miso is a living food, it is easily digestible and contains many cell-strengthening minerals. In addition to soup, there are several ways to enjoy the healthful benefits of miso, including dips, sauces, and dressings, but remember to use organic unpasteurized miso.

Soy sauce

Soy sauce is another delicious and nutritious way of getting more soy in your diet. To make sure you are getting a good quality of soy sauce to use in stir-fry or vegetable plates, see that it does not contain sugar, caramel coloring, and the dangerous food additive monosodium glutamate (MSG), which has been linked to many unhealthy reactions ranging from headaches and mild heart palpitations to death. Occasionally you will see the words "natural flavoring" or "hydrolyzed vegetable protein" on a label of soy sauce. That's the same as MSG, so don't buy it. I also always ask for no MSG at a Chinese restaurant.

Although soy sauce is a tasty addition to foods, it does not contain the same concentration of soy protein as tempeh or tofu and therefore has a more modest health benefit. Soy sauce does enhance digestion, however, while making a pleasant addition to grilled veggies, stews, beans, and dressings.

Shoyu sauce and tamari sauce

Two more additions to your meals may be natural shoyu and tamari sauce. The former adds a sweet flavor, whereas the latter has a stronger taste that comes from its higher content of glutamic acid, which is nature's MSG. We add tamari to many of our roasted vegetable and tofu dishes. Both shoyu sauce and tamari sauce are derivatives of soy.

Braggs Liquid Aminos

Braggs Liquid Aminos is a natural, non-GMO, all-purpose seasoning made from soy protein. Paul C. Bragg, America's first health food store developer, originally formulated it. Of all the liquid flavor enhancers, I favor Braggs to bring out the taste of salads (with a little olive oil), soups, veggies, rice dishes, rice and beans, stir-frys, and tempeh.

Soy cheese, soy yogurt, soy flour, and soy protein powder

There are other wonderful ways to enhance your health, longevity, and peace of mind by using tofu as a dairy substitute. Try non-GMO soy cheese, soy yogurt, soy flour, and soy protein powder. When you consume soy in any of its many varieties, you can rest assured you are doing one of the best things you can for your family's well-being and the long-term survival of the planet.

BEANS AND LEGUMES

Beans and legumes are also a nutritious and inexpensive source of low-fat protein. They contain almost no fat and are rich in fiber and good carbohydrate. Beans are avidly consumed in the healthiest diets around the world and contribute to successful aging and longevity. Better health has been noted in studies comparing Greeks eating the traditional Mediterranean diet with people having a reduced intake of beans and a greater intake of meat. This improvement does not come strictly from the elimination of meat, however. Beans have inherent health benefits because they carry a complement of phytonutrients, folic acid, and iron. They are also an important source of dietary fiber, which is associated with cardiac health.

Many people who eat meat regularly are unaware that raising animals for human consumption can be horribly depleting and polluting of our precious natural resources, including our air, water, and soil. For example, residues of animal wastes containing chemicals, drugs, and hormones have been found in surface and ground water. Another issue is global hunger. If the grain fed to animals were to be given to poor people worldwide, hunger would be significantly reduced. As you become more conscious about your food choices, you will be glad to know that selecting clean protein and alternative protein sources such as soy is not only good for your health, it helps heal our planet as well.

CHAPTER 12

The Fifth Principle: Discover Juicing and Supplements

A sure road to perfect health is to drink more and eat less. Many fruits and vegetables can be turned into a concentrated form of nutritional energy by juicing them. Raw juice, when extracted from organically grown fresh vegetables and fruits, provides the easiest way for the body to ingest a high percentage of the vitamins and minerals found in these foods. Including fresh juices in your yoga nutritional therapy program will build and regenerate your body.

Vegetable juices are usually assimilated within 10 to 15 minutes after you drink them. Actually, the concept of *drinking* your fresh vegetable juice is a misnomer. You should be chewing the juice, allowing it to mix thoroughly with your saliva. Raw juice fasts are great for losing weight and for cleansing the organs, cells, and tissues of the body. See pages 75 and 109 for more information on raw juice fasts.

Fresh juices are also alive with enzymes, which deliver vitality and energy to every cell of your body. The main benefit of juice therapy is the introduction of live foods into your body. Live food and raw food are absolutely loaded with vitamins, minerals, trace elements, and all the phytonutrients you need to send a positive healing message to your cells and genes. Recall that phytonutrients have tremendous health benefits, strengthening your immune system and cardiovascular system as well as your bones, joints, and brain. Juice therapy also promotes a healthy digestive system. Because fresh juice is predigested, it allows your digestive organs to rest, somewhat as they do during a fast. This regenerates your stomach and intestines.

In a study published in the journal *Appetite* in 2000, it was shown that drinking a glass of fresh vegetable juice before lunch removed an average of 136 calories from a meal. If you can do this a few times a day, it is possible to lose weight and also extend your life span, because fewer calories equal longer life.

Please use only fresh juice. Processed juices are dead foods, and eating or drinking them will result in low energy and recurring health problems. Following are some of the easiest juice recipes I know. They will help to get you started. If you don't have a juicer, please check the resource section to learn about the Vita-Mix juicing machine, which is the one I use and recommend.

- Carrot juice: Rich in phytonutrients, especially beta-carotene and vitamin A. Great for immune system, respiratory, and heart health. One cup of carrot juice contains the equivalent nutrition of 4 cups of raw chopped carrots.

- Carrot-beet juice: Excellent for the liver, flushing out toxins, and for strengthening the immune system.

- Carrot-celery juice: A great combination for supplying vitamin A and many important minerals. Excellent for the heart, respiratory, and immune systems.

- Cucumber juice: The best for balancing your emotions and helping you ease off substances such as alcohol, drugs, or nicotine. It is also good for skin, hair, and nails. Cucumber is a natural diuretic, which helps eliminate bloating.

- Parsley-carrot-beet-spinach-apple juice: Very energizing and healing. I like to have it at least once a week.

- Orange-carrot juice: A deliciously sweet mixture that is rich in folic acid, vitamin C, vitamin A, and potassium. Excellent as an immune system and respiratory tonic.

Juicing is a sensible, delicious, and nutritious way to immediately experience a surge in your overall health and energy. To follow my prescription "drink more, eat less," start with two 8-ounce glasses of fresh juice a day. You will notice your weight stabilize. Here is a simple way to add fresh juice to your diet.

For a complete breakfast
Drink 8 ounces of orange or pineapple juice mixed with a scoop of soy protein and ¼ scoop of green drink powder.

With lunch
Drink 8 ounces of carrot or carrot-celery juice.

With dinner
Drink 8 ounces of mixed vegetable juice. Try juicing your salad instead of eating it. Keep it simple at first, then begin to add vegetables as you get used to it. For example, take one carrot, one tomato, four slices of cucumber, four kale leaves, two sprigs of parsley, three broccoli florets, and a small pinch of alfalfa sprouts. Place them in the juicer, and you will have a great juice for energy, cancer prevention, and overall health.

When you are ready, begin to enjoy a glass of rich vegetable or fruit juice midmorning, as a snack. It's the perfect way to get your seven servings of fruits and vegetables a day and to increase your intake of fiber, vitamins, minerals, and phytonutrients.

You can even try a broccoli sprout–spinach mixture with a small amount of apple for sweetness. To prepare it, place four florets of fresh broccoli, four leaves of spinach, and half of a red apple in your juicer, and mix it up. This juice will give you a jolt of sulforaphane with its specific anticancer qualities, plus all the health-promoting enzymes and brain-protecting nutrients in spinach. Juicing can heal you and save your life.

SMOOTHIES

Another way to enjoy the many benefits of juicing is by making a smoothie, usually with fruit. Start with orange juice, grapefruit juice, and pineapple juice, then add fruit, soy protein powder, and a little ice. Mix it up—and presto, you have a very satisfying, low-calorie, nutrient-dense meal. I call this a power smoothie. There is no limit to what you can put in your smoothie. You can follow one of my recipes or design your own.

I love smoothies and usually have one for breakfast. Also, if I've been a little lax with my diet and see that a few pounds have crept on, I'll have two smoothies a day with a light dinner, and in a few days I'm back to normal.

Bliss smoothie
Blend ½ cup of orange juice, ½ cup pineapple juice, ice, and 1 scoop of vanilla soy powder. Optional: Add half a banana and two organic strawberries.

26 grams protein, 150 calories, 1 gram fat.

Benefits: stamina, decreased hunger, and mood enhancement.

*Chai freeze**
Blend ½ cup chai tea, ½ cup soy milk, and ½ to 1 cup ice.

125 calories, 1 gram fat.

Benefits: energy, mental clarity, and stamina.

*The Don Juan**·
Blend ¼ cup pineapple juice, 1 banana cut up, ¼ cup light coconut milk, ¼ cup mango, and 6 to 12 ounces ice. Drink slowly.

160 calories, 1 gram fat.

Benefit: This smoothie can ignite your libido.

Dr. Dharma's brain power drink
Blend 6 to 8 ounces vanilla soy milk, 2 scoops protein powder, ½ cup frozen blueberries, and ½ scoop green powder. You can add half an apple or half a banana as desired. Drink as the first meal of the day.

30 grams protein, 250 calories, 3 grams fat.

Benefits: enhanced physical energy and mental clarity.

*Green power**
Blend 2 ounces wheat grass juiced or ¼ to ½ scoop green drink, two or three whole dates, one banana cut up, ½ cup papaya juice, and 6 to 12 ounces ice.

240 calories, 1 gram fat

Benefits: detoxification, anti-inflammatory, and physical energy.

*Liquid sunshine**
Juice 5 carrots and ½ apple.

200 calories, 1 gram fat.

Benefits: increased energy, immune system enhancement.

*Nordine's power punch**

Blend 5 ounces skim milk, two scoops whey protein, one banana, four or five strawberries, 2 tablespoons low-fat organic yogurt, and ½ cup ice.

36 grams protein, 400 calories, 3 grams fat.

Benefits: physical strength, muscular development, endurance.

*Omega sensation**

Blend ¾ cup apple juice, one banana cut in four pieces, 1 teaspoon flaxseeds, 1 teaspoon hemp seeds, 1 teaspoon cardamom, 1 teaspoon cinnamon, and 6 to 12 ounces ice.

240 calories, 3 grams fat.

Benefits: cardiovascular health, increased energy, anti-inflammatory.

*Miraval Resort recipe.

SUPPLEMENTS AS MEDICINE

If you exist in a pristine environment, breathe perfectly clean air, drink impeccable water, eat a great diet, and either live a stress-free life or meditate a lot, you won't need to supplement your food with vitamins, minerals, or illness-specific nutrients. If you live a life other than this, you will. Occasionally I'll hear someone say that all vitamins do is produce expensive urine. I disagree. To me, expensive urine is the urine in the bedpan at a nursing home. Supplementation, as recent research shows, has the power of delaying many of the unhappy effects of aging such as immune dysfunction, heart disease, memory loss, and joint degeneration. Beyond the scientific evidence to support taking multiple vitamin and mineral tablets, there is also proof that certain nutrients are therapeutic for specific illnesses.

Many people are overfed yet undernourished. They simply don't eat well. Moreover, the food they do eat is lacking in all the important lifesaving ingredients we have been discussing in this book. There are many reasons for that. For one thing, if organic food is not used, the diet probably lacks nutrients. According to the USDA website, www.usda.gov, food has diminished in vitamin and mineral content by as much as 50 percent or more over the past twenty-five to thirty years. For example, between 1963 and 2000, the vitamin C content of spinach dropped by 45 percent. Since 1975, the calcium in broccoli has fallen by 50 percent, and the iron in watercress has plummeted by 88 percent. The National Academy of Sciences has issued an alert to warn us that it now takes twice as many vegetables as was previously thought to give the daily requirement of vitamin A.

This is a critical situation. A recent summary of research published by the Life Extension Foundation highlights the grave danger:

- 90 percent of women and 71 percent of men get less than the RDA for vitamin B_6.
- Men with the lowest amount of vitamin C have a 62 percent increased risk of cancer and a 57 percent increased risk of dying from any cause.
- People with low levels of beta-carotene, vitamin E, and selenium are more likely to get cancer.
- The area of China with the lowest micronutrient intake has the highest cancer rate. Supplementation lowers the rate.
- American children have inadequate levels of vitamin E.

Before implementing the yoga nutritional therapy program, most of my patients were not even getting seven to nine servings of fruits and vegetables a day. (A serving is 1 cup of a raw vegetable, ½ cup of a cooked vegetable, or 8 ounces of fresh juice.) Because of that, many of them were nutrient deficient.

I now routinely prescribe supplements to my patients. And it works. A person's response to supplementation can be quite dramatic. Many people who are experiencing a diverse range of symptoms notice an immediate boost in their well-being, energy, and happiness. Beyond that, when used as part of an integrative medical program, supplemental nutrients can reverse many medical conditions.

Although many conventional practitioners still don't support their use, the general public does not hesitate to spend its hard-earned money on dietary supplements. National surveys show that close to 50 percent of Americans take some form of supplement. The U.S. Food and Drug Administration estimates that more than 29,000 different such products are on the market. According to the *National Business Journal,* sales of supplements reached $14 billion in 1998, up from $8 billion just four years earlier. People are not going to waste billions of dollars on something that doesn't work.

Many people take supplements without knowing exactly what they're doing. Understanding how to use nutrients as medicine is crucial to living long and well. Some patients I see are under-dosing. They're not getting enough of whatever it is they need to take. One reason is that the RDAs—the Recommended Daily Allowances as determined by the U.S. Government—are just too low for maximal health. The RDA is the *minimum* amount of that nutrient you need to stay alive. If you are in search of anti-aging, maximum health, and longevity, the RDAs are simply insufficient.

Here's another problem: even many physician-authors suggest doses that are not high enough. Again, I believe this is because they lack the clinical expertise and advanced study that many leading-edge physicians possess. Some of the doctors I consider to be at the vanguard are Julian Whitaker, M.D., of the Whitaker Wellness Institute; David Leonardi, M.D., of Cenegenics Life Enhancement Center; and Stephen T. Sinatra, M.D., of Optimum Health Institute. In addition, the well-researched suggestions of the Life Extension Foundation are also instrumental in formulating the clinically effective supplement program I use regularly.

Each and every vitamin and mineral is important. There are also some newly discovered antioxidant combinations that are crucial for specific bodily functions, such as coenzyme Q10 for increased energy production and N-acetylcysteine to reduce incidence of the flu. Also, it has recently been shown that there are illness-specific supplements. For example, we now know of specific nutrients to slow brain aging and reverse signs of memory loss, including Alzheimer's disease. They include the antioxidant vitamin E, the supplement phosphatidylserine, and the herb gingko biloba.

ANTIOXIDANT COMBINATIONS

One of the most important advances in vitamin therapy is the use of new and advanced antioxidant combinations. This is important because antioxidants fight free radicals, which are highly unstable molecules that seek out and destroy normal cells in your body. Free radicals are thought to play a major role in the development of brain aging, heart disease, cancer, fatigue, chronic pain, and immune system dysfunction. By age twenty-seven, the rate of free-radical damage outpaces your natural ability to repair it. Therefore, adopting a potent vitamin therapy will saturate every cell in your body with life-saving antioxidants and immune system–stimulating nutrients.

This is not just theory. In a 1999 study published in *Lancet*, hypertensive patients taking only 500 mg of the antioxidant vitamin C had a significant drop in their blood pressure. Taking 800 IU of vitamin E (d-alpha-tocopherol), 2,000 patients lowered their risk of heart attack by 77 percent, according to an analysis published in *Current Opinion in Lipidology.* Hepatitis C has reportedly been cured with an antioxidant cocktail of 600 mg of alpha-lipoic acid, 400 mcg of selenium, and 900 mg of silymarin. In a 2000 study published in the *Journal of the National Cancer Institute,* 631 subjects with precancerous changes in their stomach taking 1,200 mcg of selenium were five times as likely as those taking placebo to have a reversal of their condition.

NEW ANTIOXIDANT COMBINATIONS

Some newer supplements actually hunt down free radicals inside the mitochondria, the energy power plants within each cell. Others protect your genes, allowing them to communicate signals of health and healing to the rest of your body. Of course, vitamins C and E and the minerals zinc and selenium are well-known antioxidants. Here is a short list of the newest discoveries in antioxidants that you need to know about:

Alpha-lipoic acid

Alpha-lipoic acid is an energy-producing antioxidant, helping your body regenerate other antioxidants such as vitamins E and C. Preliminary work suggests that it may be very effective in the fight against heart disease. Alpha-lipoic acid is a great free radical scavenger. I prescribe a dose of 250 mg to help promote successful aging. Preliminary research, however, suggests amounts as high as 1,000 mg for AIDS and other life-threatening diseases.

Coenzyme Q10

This energy-producing substance has been the subject of many published medical reports, articles, and books. Coenzyme Q10 is so powerful that it has helped some patients eliminate the need for heart transplant surgery. A colleague of mine, after hearing about coenzyme Q10 at a medical conference, returned to work and prescribed the compound for three of his sickest heart patients. All three improved dramatically, going from invalid status to being able to walk. Two of the three no longer needed their oxygen tanks.

I first heard about coenzyme Q10 while attending a conference on Alzheimer's disease. I asked a presenter if he thought everyone should be taking it. He said to me very seriously, "Dharma, they should put it in the drinking water." Coenzyme Q10 is an excellent metabolic enhancer and free radical scavenger. I recommend doses of 100 to 300 mg per day. Although it costs a bit more than other supplements, I believe the literature shows that it's worth the money. Because it is costly, some formulations include only a fraction of the proper dose—say, only 30 mg. In my opinion, you are better off taking coenzyme Q10 less often at the right dose than taking it regularly in an ineffective amount.

Glutathione

Glutathione is the body's master antioxidant. Many researchers consider it to be the most important one. It is synthesized in our cells to fight off the effects of metabolism, which can age us and disrupt our DNA, leading to cancer. Glutathione plays a vital role in liver health and is especially helpful in the detoxification of drugs and pollutants. Experts on antioxidants believe that glutathione is essential for a strong immune system. However, it cannot be taken by mouth because it is not absorbed from the digestive system.

Taking alpha-lipoic acid is the best way to augment your glutathione production, but there is one exception. In recent clinical work, David Perlmutter, M.D., of the Permutter Health Center in Florida, and I have shown that glutathione, when injected intravenously, can help reverse the symptoms of Parkinson's disease. If I had Parkinson's, I would not hesitate to try this therapy.

Indole-3-carbinol

Indole-3-carbinol (I-3-C), a phytonutrient found in cruciferous vegetables such as cabbage, is an antioxidant and cancer fighter. According to the Life Extension Foundation, medical research on I-3-C dates back to the 1960s.

How does I-3-C fight cancer? First, it actually promotes cancer cell death. Then, it prevents DNA damage, blocks the negative effects of estrogen, and stops the growth of prostate cancer cells. Published reports also indicate that I-3-C may prevent cancers resulting from pesticides and other chemicals. Moreover, I-C-3 inhibits the growth of human breast cancer cells better than the estrogen-blocking drug tamoxifen by 30 percent.

Do you need an I-C-3 supplement if you eat my seven to nine servings of vegetables daily? Probably not. If there is doubt, however, I'd say to use the supplement. It can't hurt you and may help you prevent the development of cancer. The suggested dose is 200 mg twice a day for women and 200 mg three times a day for men.

N-acetylcysteine

N-acetylcysteine is a derivative of the sulfur-containing amino acid cysteine. A 1997 trial published in *European Respiratory Journal* showed that 600 mg markedly reduced incidence of the flu. N-acetylcysteine is converted in the body to glutathione, one of our most important naturally occurring antioxidants. It has been reported to increase survival in HIV/AIDS patients. It is a powerful addition to our armamentarium. The recommended dose is generally 250 to 600 mg.

Vitamin B_{12} and folic acid

These two nutrients are critically important because of the role they play in controlling homocysteine. If your level of homocysteine is high, your chances of developing heart disease and memory loss are increased. The correct dose for vitamin B_{12} is 100 to 150 mcg a day. For folic acid it is 400 to 800 mcg a day.

NEW THERAPEUTIC SUPPLEMENTS
AND SUPPLEMENT COMBINATIONS

Three types of supplements—multivitamins, the mineral zinc, and various antioxidants—have been shown to delay the diminished vision many people experience with age. One of my healing partners, a seventy-four-year-old retired lawyer, had a scary time recently when he flew into a West Coast city for the first time, arrived at dusk, and had to rent a car to drive up to the northern part of the state. He was shocked that he had such difficulty seeing at night in an unfamiliar location. His doctor diagnosed an early form of macular degeneration, the most common type of age-related vision loss.

I told him about a study published by Dr. Emily Chew, Director of the Epidemiology and Clinical Research at the National Eye Institute, part of the National Institutes of Health (NIH). The research, published in *Archives of Ophthalmology* in 2000, examined the impact of supplements on the vision of 3,600 people aged 55 to 80. It showed a very positive effect in stemming visual deterioration. The doses used were 500 mg of vitamin C, 400 IU of vitamin E, 15 mg of beta-carotene, 80 mg of zinc oxide, and 2 mg of cupric oxide, a form of copper that complements zinc. Dr. Chew's research is one example of the positive synergistic effect of taking proper doses of antioxidant supplements. Adding the phytonutrient bilberry, found naturally in berries or in supplemental form, may augment this effect for night vision.

OTHER IMPORTANT NEW THERAPEUTIC SUPPLEMENTS
DHEA

Dehydroepiandrosterone (DHEA) is not actually new. In fact, I have written about its many benefits in two other books. However, I must discuss

DHEA again because many people still do not know about its multiple clinical benefits. Additionally, it seems that even some physician writers are unaware of the mounting scientific evidence of DHEA's benefits.

DHEA is a weak steroid released by the adrenal gland in men and women. It is the most abundant steroid hormone in the human body. Low levels of it are associated with aging and disease. I measure the blood DHEA level routinely on my patients and have noticed it to be low in nearly everyone who has age-related loss of mental function. Low DHEA levels have also been found to correlate with immune dysfunction, inflammation, increased risk of some cancers, more heart disease in men, and osteoporosis. Research by Samuel Yen, M.D., of the University of California San Diego Medical Center has shown that DHEA is a mild mood enhancer. It also plays a valuable role as part of the body's antioxidant defense system. For more information on DHEA, turn to pages 163 and 169.

MGN3

An extract of rice bran and mushroom, MGN3 has been clinically shown to help patients fight cancer. It triples natural killer cell activity, which is crucial in recovery from cancer and in maintaining health in HIV/AIDS. MGN3 has also been shown to enhance the activity of B cells, important to the immune system, and to increase the levels of interferon, another important immune-enhancing substance. This means it is a powerful immune system stimulator. For more information on MGN3, please turn to page 193.

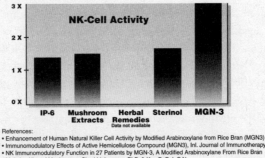

References:
• Enhancement of Human Natural Killer Cell Activity by Modified Arabinoxylane from Rice Bran (MGN3)
• Immunomodulatory Effects of Active Hemicellulose Compound (MGN3), Inl. Journal of Immunotherapy
• NK Immunomodulatory Function in 27 Patients by MGN-3, A Modified Arabinoxylane From Rice Bran
• Maitake, King of Mushrooms, Shari Lieberman, PhD. & Ken BaBal, C.N.
• Published Advertisements 1998, (Inositol + IP-6)
• Esslac–Published Data Re: NK-Cell Proliferation-Not Found
• PSK–Published Data Re: NK-Cell Proliferation-Not Found
• Floressence, Published Data Re: NK-Cell Proliferation-Not Found

Courtesy of Lane Labs, Allendale, NJ

Mistletoe (Iscador)

This is a controversial cancer fighter. It became notorious when one of its main proponents, actress Suzanne Somers, discussed it on *Larry King Live* in 2001. She said she was taking mistletoe extract after undergoing lumpectomy and radiation therapy for breast cancer. Of course, many in the conventional medical establishment were among the first to classify it as quackery. What they apparently didn't know was that this botanical, plus standard treatment, helps cancer patients live 40 percent longer.

Scientific evidence showing the effectiveness of using mistletoe to aid healing and longevity in cancer patients was published in the May 2001 issue of *Alternative Therapies in Health and Medicine,* the leading journal on integrative medicine. The article, by Dr. Ronald Grossarth-Maticek, described a study whose results showed that breast cancer patients receiving conventional treatment plus mistletoe survived 40 percent longer than those who received the usual therapy alone. Mistletoe is currently the most widely used cancer drug in Germany.

Mistletoe is generally administered by injection beneath the skin, sometimes intravenously, and sometimes near the tumor. Rudolf Steiner, the founder of anthroposophical medicine, a medical system that uses herbal and homeopathic medicines, first used it in the 1930s for cancer therapy. The use of mistletoe as a complementary therapy is indicated for cancers of the breast, colon, rectum, or lung, but not for leukemia or lymphoma. Mistletoe is a very promising treatment for cancer, and we look forward to more research on its benefits and contraindications.

Perilla oil

This oil is an especially potent source of alpha-linolenic acid (ALA), which is the primary active ingredient in flaxseed oil. There have been reports of striking reductions in mortality among people who consume ALA. Perilla oil, with its high content of ALA, lowers the risk of heart disease in a matter of weeks. It also reduces the risk of breast and colon cancer. This oil, rich in omega-3 fatty acids, significantly inhibits inflammatory cytokines, which are linked to alarm illnesses such as rheumatoid arthritis, colitis, atherosclerosis, and a host of autoimmune and age-related illnesses.

If you are a strict vegetarian who isn't taking enough flax oil, or if you're not eating enough salmon, perilla oil is a good supplement. My recommendation is to start off with six 1,000-mg capsules daily, which provides enough ALA for your body to reap the benefits of healthful omega-3 fatty acids.

SAM-e

SAM-e (S-adenosylmethionine) is a very popular antidepressant. A pilot study in the November 2000 edition of the journal *Movement Disorders* showed that it was highly effective in alleviating the symptoms of depression in patients with Parkinson's disease. What made this study even more significant was that the patients had not improved when they took conventional antidepressant medications, such as Prozac.

An exciting report from Germany indicated that SAM-e may also protect against brain aging, at least in rodents. The study found that SAM-e increased glutathione levels by 50 percent, increased antioxidant activity by 98 percent, and decreased free radical activity by 46 percent.

To alleviate symptoms of depression, most studies show that doses of 800 mg to 1,600 mg a day are required for three weeks. For anti-aging effects, 300 mg to 900 mg can be taken. There are no reported side effects.

RECOMMENDED AMOUNTS OF DAILY VITAMINS

Here are the amounts of vitamins I recommend to my patients. It's also the regimen I take myself. To insure you are getting a strong enough multivitamin, make sure it contains at least 50 mg of vitamin B complex. If so, it usually contains an appropriate amount of other recommended ingredients as well.

Vitamin A (beta-carotene and mixed carotenoids): 10,000 to 15,000 units
Function: protects cell membranes and DNA

Vitamin C: 1500 to 3,000 mg
Function: immune system, connective tissue, and blood vessels

Vitamin D: 600 IU
Function: healthy bones and calcium intake

Vitamin E (d-alpha-tocopherol): 800 IU
Function: heart, immune system, and free radical fighter

Other vitamins
B$_1$ (thiamine): 50 mg
Function: energy

B$_2$ (riboflavin): 50 mg
Function: vision and cells

B$_3$ (niacin and niacinamide): 50 mg each
Function: cardiovascular health and cholesterol lowering

B$_6$ (pyridoxine): 50 mg
Function: brain, nerves, and immune system

Folate (folic acid): 800 mcg
Function: heart and brain protection, homocysteine regulation

B$_{12}$ (cyanocobalamin): 150 mcg
Function: nerves, blood, homocysteine metabolism

Biotin: 50 mcg
Function: energy, healthy hair and bones

Pantothenic acid: 50 mg
Function: energy, combats ill effects of stress

Para-aminobenzoic acid (PABA): 50 mg
Function: overall health

Minerals
Calcium: 1,000 mg
Function: nerves, cells, bones, energy

Chromium: 200 mcg
Function: glucose metabolism, energy, heart, cholesterol reduction

Copper: 2 mg
Function: nerves, cells

Iodine: 200 mcg
Function: energy

Magnesium: 500 mg
Function: heart, blood pressure, energy, muscle relaxation

Manganese: 10 mg
Function: energy, glucose metabolism

Molybdenum: 200 mcg
Function: energy
Potassium: 60 mg
Function: energy

Selenium: 200 mcg
Function: cell health, antioxidant, cancer prevention

Zinc: 30 mg
Function: antioxidant, prostate, eyes, immunity

Other important substances
Betaine hydrochloride: 50 mg
Function: digestion

Boron: 10 mcg
Function: hair, energy

Choline: 10 mg
Function: brain, liver, and nerve function

Citrus bioflavonoids: 100 mg
Function: immunity, blood vessels, connective tissue

Green tea extract: 50 mg
Function: cancer prevention

Hesperedin bioflavonoid complex: 100 mg
Function: immunity, blood vessels, connective tissue

Inositol: 10 mg
Function: brain and nerve function

Silicon: 100 mg
Function: every system

Trimethylglycine: 50 mg
Function: metabolism

Vanadium: 50 mg
Function: energy, many bodily systems

VITAMINS AND MINERALS IN FOODS

Supplements are important, but whenever you can you should eat these very low-alarm foods so that you'll get their vitamins and minerals directly. Remember to go organic.

Vitamin A: Apples, bananas (including the white "strings" inside the peel), carrots, papaya, oranges.

Vitamin B: Apples, coconuts, papayas.

Vitamin C: Apples, carrots, coconut milk, grapes, green chilies, kiwi, lemons, olives, oranges, papaya.

Calcium: Apples, bananas, broccoli, cabbage, carrots, dairy (such as low-fat yogurt), figs, kale, lemons, oranges, papaya, parsley, sesame seeds, spinach, watercress.

Vitamin D: Papaya.

Vitamin E: Sunflower seeds.

Iodine: Coconut.

Iron: Apples, apricots, bananas, parsley.

Lecithin: Sesame seeds.

Magnesium: Apples, coconuts, grapes, lemons, oranges, sesame seeds.

Phosphorus: Bananas (very high), coconuts, olives, red chilies.

Potassium: Apples, bananas, coconut, grapes, horseradish, lemons, olives, oranges, parsley, zucchini.

Protein: Coconut is a complete protein.

Sodium: Apples, bananas, oranges.

Sulfur: Chili peppers, garlic, horseradish, onions, parsley, watercress.

Zinc: Sunflower seeds.

CHAPTER 13

The Sixth Principle:
Cook Consciously and Eat Mindfully

Mealtimes can be an oasis of comfort and healing—or quite the opposite. When Kirti and I first married, our only domestic tension concerned my eating habits. Being your typical American doctor, I ate fast. I perfected this skill as a young intern and resident in anesthesiology, when I didn't have time to sit down to eat. This was especially true when I was on call at the San Francisco General Hospital Trauma Unit. I just gulped food down as fast as I could, usually at midnight. Fifteen years later, this was not a good practice to bring into a marriage with a woman used to celebrating mealtimes. I have made the effort to change, and although I occasionally creep back into my old ways of stressful eating, I am happy to report that our meals are now usually peaceful.

Unfortunately, many people today eat at the same breakneck speed they use for everything else. You may even be frustrated or angry when it's mealtime. If you are anxious, depressed, or distracted when eating, your body will not assimilate food well, and you will not receive the nourishment you need. It is vitally important to actively switch on your own inner healing state, especially if you usually eat while watching television news, discussing business, or doing other potentially upsetting things. With a little bit of conscious effort, you can create a divine space in which to enjoy your food. One way I've found to slow down my rhythm is to take a few deep breaths before dining. Another way is to say a prayer. The purpose of blessing your food is to express reverence for the presence of God in everything. I do that by chanting "Sat Nam" three times. "Sat Nam" is a healing sound, or mantra, which reminds me that food is a gift from our Creator.

Many lifestyles and religions have similar techniques. Jewish people say a prayer thanking God for the bread of the earth, and Christians pray in the name of Jesus to bless the food. I have many patients and friends who, although they aren't religious, stop for a moment to give thanks before eating. It's a very nice thing to do and has a beneficial effect on your digestion.

By opening your heart and showing gratitude for your food, you are bowing your head in reverence to the King of Kings, the One, the Giver who encompasses all of nature: wind, sun, sky, and earth, all of which came together to grant you sustenance. This simple act supports your quest for maximum health.

Here are examples of other blessings:

Buddhist: On this plate, I see the entire Cosmos supporting my sustenance.

Christian: In the name of Jesus, we pray that we may be blessed by this food. That it nurture us and sustain us. Amen.

Hindu: All things come from God, and all things go to God. We worship the Divine in food.

Jewish: Blessed art Thou, O Lord our God, Creator of the Universe, who brings forth bread from the earth.

Sikh: May this food remind us of the blessings of the Guru. May the grace of the Guru lead us to the infinity of wisdom, prosperity, and health. Sat Nam.

Sufi: Come and eat with us even if you have broken your vows a hundred times. Come, come again, come. God is great.

Now that you have blessed your food, you're ready to eat it. Take a good whiff of it to prepare your salivary secretions. It's good to take your time chewing your food, too. In yoga nutritional therapy, as in Chinese medicine, it is recommended to chew your food until it is almost in a liquid state. This markedly improves your digestion because the enzymes have ample time to be released from your pancreas and other organs and to get to your stomach and small intestine. Let the food linger in your mouth. Really feel the textures of your food, and taste the tastes. Occasionally, eat totally in silence and see the difference that makes in your appreciation of the wonderful gift of food.

COOK CONSCIOUSLY

Actually, healing with food should begin even before the food arrives at the table. We must be alert and mindful about what we eat, and that begins with the choices made at the store. Choices begin in your mind. If you can, take a moment to do the following:

- Meditate, or clear your mind with a few deep breaths, before entering the market. This will also help you buy the right things for you and your family while not reacting emotionally to subliminal messages that are implanted in your mind by advertising.
- Another option is to make a list in a relaxed state before embarking on a trip to the store. Food provides vital energy for the body while creating subtle energy for your spirit. If you are frenetic when shopping, you will make the wrong choices.
- Before shopping, you might find it useful to refer back to your food log exercises, such as shopping by color. Remember to have your shopping cart look like a rainbow of nutrition.
- Experiment by trying something new—perhaps try a more exotic food such as goat's milk, baked tofu, or miso soup.

A conscious cook is always aware that every body is a temple of God and that to maintain the health, purity, and strength that are worthy of the soul, only wholesome, cleansing, and nutritious foods should be eaten. Nervous vibrations at mealtime may negate the health outcomes you seek by using food as medicine. When you are ready to prepare the meal, create a peaceful space by singing a joyful song, chanting an uplifting mantra, or listening to beautiful music. The cook should create a positive, blissful feeling, which brings happiness and love into the eating experience.

The need to hurry while preparing food has caused an overreliance on the microwave oven. While I don't deny that it can be a convenience, I also think microwaves probably can change the molecular configuration of food and reduce its vital energy. When you institute a natural healing program using pure foods, rich in nature's own phytonutrients, I suggest using the microwave as little as possible and keeping your distance from it as it cooks, just in case it emits dangerous levels of electromagnetic energy. I strongly recommened you use a microwave oven only for heating food quickly, not for cooking that takes more than a few minutes.

Cooking consciously and eating mindfully allow us to remember that everything we eat comes from God, as do our health and healing. Dining will become a deeply spiritual experience, and eating in consciousness will allow you to truly heal.

CHAPTER 14

The Seventh Principle:
Make the Transition

Many Americans eat more animal foods in their lifetime than contained on an entire Iowa farm. If you consume the standard American diet throughout your life, you will have eaten the equivalent of eleven cows, four veal calves, three lambs, forty-three pigs, one thousand chickens, forty-five turkeys, and eight hundred fish. Science has shown that this type of diet is detrimental to your health and, in large measure, is responsible for the epidemics of heart disease, cancer, and other degenerative diseases we have today.

By contrast, studies of vegetarian populations—Seventh Day Adventists, Mormons, and nonreligious groups—have shown that major diseases occur markedly less. For instance, Mormons, who characteristically eat little meat, have 50 percent less cancer than the US population. Beginning in 1983, Dean Ornish, M.D., has shown that patients with significant heart disease who consumed a vegetarian diet displayed a complete reduction of plaque in their coronary arteries. The *New England Journal of Medicine,* moreover, reported in a 2001 study of 88,000 women that those who ate the most animal fat were nearly twice as likely to develop colon cancer as those who ate the least.

For these reasons and others we have discussed throughout this book, the yoga nutritional therapy program is a continuum moving toward a plant-based diet. Wherever you are on the continuum at this moment is fine; it's just a starting point. We begin where you are now and aim in the direction of a diet free of red meat and high in organic vegetables, fruits, and some grains. If you make it that far, I will be delighted and you will be infinitely healthier. If you take the next step and eliminate fish, chicken, and eggs—that is, become a lacto-vegetarian (a little dairy is okay)—I will be ecstatic and so will you.

Whatever you decide, I believe you must make long-term decisions so that your transition will last. Personal styles differ in people aiming to achieve the goal of a plant-based diet. Some folks can make it happen overnight. Others need months or perhaps even years to get there. If, however, you already have a significant illness, the faster you make the change to a yoga nutritional therapy diet, the quicker you will be on the road to healing.

The YNT program, for very practical reasons, bases food selection on your lifestyle choices, vegetarian or not. It provides the foundation for you to build upon. YNT, therefore, is a flexible transitional system for you to use as you strive for the best possible health. All my healing partners lie somewhere between strict vegetarianism and the standard American diet and between very active and sedentary life styles. The program is diverse enough to accommodate them all.

The yoga nutritional therapy approach allows plenty of protein—as high as 40 percent of total calories depending on your activity level—but limits the amount you get from animals. Low-fat meat substitutes and protein powders from soy and whey are additional sources of protein to add to your diet. Soy, for example, is 43 percent protein.

Among the chief complaints expressed by many of my patients is fatigue. The yoga nutritional therapy diet will create more energy for you to direct toward enjoying life and healing. Saturated fat sources of protein such as red meat and eggs require more energy to digest than they often impart to the healing system of the body. They also plug up elimination and retard immunity. A vegetarian diet requires less energy than a standard diet to digest, supplies more nutrients, and supports your vital life force. Because animal products are high-frequency alarm foods, eating meat makes it harder to concentrate and be productive. By following a plant-based diet, you will find that you have improved focus and higher productivity in your daily life.

DETERMINING YOUR ENERGY NEEDS

How many calories do you need? Multiply your current weight in pounds by 10 for women and 11 for men, i.e., 135 pounds $\times$ 10 = 1,350 calories for your basic needs.

Next, figure your energy needs for physical activity. Determine which of the following activity levels most closely matches your lifestyle:

10 percent—sedentary: mainly sitting, driving, lying down, sleeping, standing, reading, typing, or other low-intensity activities.

20 percent—light activity: light exercise, such as walking for no more than two hours a day.

30 percent—moderate activity: moderate exercise three to five times per week, such as heavy housework, gardening, and dancing.

40 percent—much activity: active physical sports or labor-intensive job.

Then, multiply your basic energy needs by your activity level. If one 135-pound woman has a moderately active lifestyle, the equation would look like this:

$$1,350 \times 30 \text{ percent} = 405 \text{ calories}$$

Next, multiply by 10 percent for calories needed for digestion and absorption of nutrients:

$$1,350 + 405 = 1,755 \times 10 \text{ percent} = 175.5 + 1,755 = 1,930.5 \text{ calories}$$

Her total energy needs demand 1,930.5 calories per day.

If you desire or need to lose weight, subtract 500 calories per day from your total, and you will lose 1 pound a week.

ESTABLISHING YOUR FOOD PREFERENCES

In this interactive section, list your food preferences. Becoming clear about your favorite foods may require some thoughtful awareness, but many of my healing partners have told me that this exercise helped them gain important insights into their eating habits. This awareness will allow you to establish healthy eating as a lifestyle choice rather than resort to a fad diet.

Category	Likes	Dislikes	Usual Intake
Protein/dairy			
Starches			
Grains			
Cereals			
Starchy veggies			
Beans			
Fruit			
Vegetables			
Fat/other			
Snacks			
Your comments			

SNACKS

I've found that some people don't pay attention to their snacks. Having a wholesome snack during the day helps reduce hunger. If you need more protein, a smoothie with soy or whey powder helps. If you need fruit, have an apple. And don't forget to drink eight glasses of pure water every day.

CUTTING THOSE 500 CALORIES PER DAY

By cutting back about 500 calories per day, you will lose 1 pound a week. If you are exercising, you will become leaner and have stronger muscles to go with that weight loss. When you do this, you are practicing mild caloric restriction, which is life extending.

The easiest way to cut back on calories is to reduce your portion size to the amount listed at the end of this chapter and in Appendix B. You don't necessarily have to worry about counting every calorie, but you do have to use good common sense in choosing how much you eat.

Remember to exercise four times a week, drink eight glasses of pure water every day, and meditate to stay calm, focused, and in the moment. If you are present in your body, you will naturally discover the correct portion size for you.

Once you reach your ideal body weight, you can reintroduce about 500 healthy calories per day to maintain it.

Recall that the key to the YNT program, in addition to using nonmeat sources for protein, is to include at least seven servings of veggies and fruits per day. One vegetable serving is only half a cup of cooked or raw vegetables and a whole cup of raw leafy greens, such as romaine lettuce or spinach. One fruit serving is one medium piece or half a cup of cooked or raw fruit, a quarter cup of dried fruit, or 6 ounces (¾ cup) of fruit juice. See Appendix B for a complete portion and calorie list for all foods.

If you eat red meat, limit your portion to three 3-ounce cooked servings (about the size of a deck of cards) per week. Use your meat as a side dish rather than a main course. For example, instead of a roast beef sandwich, top off a plate of grilled vegetables with a thin slice of roast beef.

SOME FINAL TIPS ON MAKING THE TRANSITION TO A YOGA NUTRITIONAL THERAPY PROGRAM

- Begin substituting nonmeat protein sources immediately to ensure that you get enough protein without the fat. The following meal plan will show you how. Refer to Appendix C for a list of nonmeat protein products.
- Always keep a protein bar, an apple, or your favorite fruit on hand for a snack.

- Consider taking a class in vegetarian cooking or buying a vegetarian cookbook. I've listed a few of my favorite vegetarian cookbooks in Appendix E, Resources. You can also learn a lot about healthful cooking from various cable television shows.
- Try something new each time you go shopping. Pick up a whole grain, like quinoa, that you've never tried before.
- Add low-calorie flavor enhancers to your salads: a ripe juicy tomato, baby carrots, or sprouts. Use olive oil and Braggs Liquid Aminos as a salad dressing, and pass up the high-calorie cheese, croutons, or bacon bits.
- When dining out, go meatless. Try an ethnic restaurant with plant-based entrees.
- Have a Mediterranean dessert. Try a fruit such as apple, melon, or pineapple, or make a fruit salad. It's delicious and satisfies your sweet tooth without all the fat, sugar, and calories.
- Eat breakfast.

PUTTING IT ALL TOGETHER

Now that you have the list of your food preferences, and you have identified the foods that you will be increasing or decreasing, it's time to put it all together and make the transition.

Here is a sample meal plan that will help you structure your food intake. Of course, you can substitute items with your favorite foods, but keep in mind that you want to keep a balance between your calories, carbohydrates, protein, and fat.

SAMPLE MEAL PLAN

Breakfast
1 cup of fruit with ½ cup low fat yogurt, 1 slice of dry whole-wheat toast, 8 oz. of juice, tea (green or black), or coffee (Decaf is best).
or
1 cup oatmeal with ½ cup low-fat organic cottage cheese, 1 fresh fruit, or 1 cup cubed fruit, or 6 oz. juice, 1 cup tea (green or black) or coffee.
or

1 cup protein smoothie (see page 111 for recipes).
or
3- egg-white omelet with spinach, tomato, and onion; 1 slice dry nine-grain toast; 6 oz. juice; 1 cup tea (green or black) or coffee.
With breakfast, take your supplements. See page 120 for recommended doses.

Midmorning snack
1 cup protein smoothie, if you didn't already have one for breakfast.
or
1 Protein bar.
or
1 fresh fruit, if you had a high-protein breakfast.

Lunch
3–5 oz. tofu or chicken, 1½ cup mung beans (or other bean), plus ½ cup rice, or 1 cup millet or other grain stew.
2–3 cups green or mixed salad, or 1½ cup other vegetables, cooked.
1 whole-wheat pita bread or tortilla, or 1 slice of nine-grain bread, if you haven't already had it for breakfast.

Midafternoon snack
8 oz. fresh vegetable juice.
or
8 oz. of a protein smoothie.
or
1 protein bar.
or
Almond or tahini butter and jelly sandwich: 2 tablespoons of either nut butter, 1 tablespoon of jelly.

Dinner
3–5 oz. Salmon, 5 oz. soy in the form of tempeh or tofu; or 1 veggie burger.
½ cup brown rice, cooked.

1½–3 cups vegetables, steamed, stir-fried, or baked.
1 fruit for dessert.

Evening snack
Celery with nonfat dip.
or
1 cup apple crisp.
or
½–1 cup low fat yogurt.

Let's review portion size again to be sure you understand it.

Each *protein* serving should be the size of a deck of cards.

Each *vegetable* or *fruit* serving should be the size of a medium apple.

Your *fat* serving per meal should be ½ tablespoon of good fat, such as extra virgin olive oil, flaxseed oil, or ghee (clarified butter).

Use your intuition to choose from the options on the sample daily menu. Be creative, and add as much variety as you can.

FOOD LOG EXERCISE #10

To gain the wisdom and healing power of whole, natural foods, try this visualization exercise followed by the suggested practice. Find a quiet place to sit, and have your food log and a pencil handy.

Come to a comfortable seated position. Inhale and exhale through your nose a few times, and allow yourself to completely relax. In your mind's eye, focus on your typical dinner plate. Visualize what you eat on an average day. Perhaps you have already started to make a few changes since beginning this book and participating in the previous exercises. Visualize your plate as it is now.

Is your plate mostly covered by an animal protein such as red meat, or do vegetables take up most of the plate? Notice the colors. Smell the aromas. Feel the texture of the food in your mouth, and taste the flavors. Is your plate absolutely healthful, or is there room for improvement? Meditate on the changes you would like to incorporate into your plate to make it a perfectly healthful one, based on what you have read thus far and what you know from prior experience.

Now, inhale through your nose, hold your breath for a moment or so, and let the breath go out easily through your nose. Drift into an even more relaxed state of mind. Now visualize the perfect plate for you. Perhaps it will contain soy, for protein, in the form of tofu or a soy burger. Or, if you eat meat, see only a small portion of chicken or fish and a larger amount of fresh, raw, or slightly steamed vegetables. Visualize all the colors. See the orange of carrot, the red of beets, the dark green of kale, the pale green of broccoli, and the off-white of cauliflower. What colors are on your ideal plate? Visualize a small portion of grains—perhaps a bed of fluffy brown rice with sliced mixed vegetables. Finally, as you sit, still very relaxed, see the size of your portions becoming appropriate to your physical activity level.

When you've let this picture of your perfect plate sink into your mind and it feels easy, peaceful, and effortless there, take a deep breath. Hold the breath as you stretch your arms up above your head, and then lower them as you exhale through your nose and relax. Enjoy the new awareness of your perfect plate.

Now it's time to take that awareness into your life. In your food log, draw your current dinner plate and your ideal plate. Then compare your plates with the drawings below. See where your current diet fits. Think back to your visualization of the optimal diet for you. Is it closer to plate 1 (the Piscean plate), plate 2 (the transitional plate), or the Aquarian plate (plate 3)?

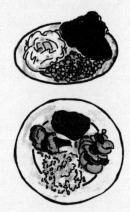

Plate 1
The Piscean Plate

Plate 2
The Transitional Plate

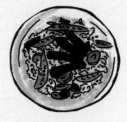

Plate 3
The Aquarian Plate

Using the sample menu on pages 133 through 135, begin the process of trying to make your actual plate resemble your ideal plate as often as possible.

HARI'S PERFECT PLATE

Hari, my daughter, is a specialist in natural therapeutics and an expert in organic food preparation. Following is a wonderful recipe for Hari's perfect plate:

Salad
Makes 4 servings

4 cups mixed greens
2 tablespoons mixed raw nuts
2 tablespoons raisins
1 cup baked tofu, chopped

DRESSING:
3 teaspoons extra virgin olive oil
¼ cup orange juice
2 teaspoons Braggs Liquid Aminos

Toss the salad in a mixing bowl. In a separate bowl, whisk all the dressing ingredients. Toss salad with dressing, and serve.

Main course: Spinach Surprise
Makes 4 servings

2 teaspoons extra virgin olive oil
3 cloves garlic, minced

3 green onions, chopped
1 cup mushrooms, chopped
2 bunches spinach
¼ teaspoon sea salt
¼ teaspoon pepper
2 tablespoons lemon juice
1½ tablespoon grated romano or parmesan cheese

Lightly cover a skillet with olive oil. Saute garlic, green onions, and mushrooms for 5 minutes. Fill skillet with thoroughly washed and chopped spinach. Add salt, pepper, and lemon juice. Cook with lid on for 2 to 3 minutes. Sprinkle grated romano or parmesan cheese on top, and serve.

Delicious, nutritious beverage: Yogi Tea

For each cup of tea, begin with 10 ounces of water. Bring the water to a rapid boil, and add (for each cup):

4 whole black peppercorns
4 whole green cardamom pods
3 whole cloves
½ stick cinnamon
½ inch slice fresh gingerroot

Cover and let boil for 15 to 20 minutes. Then add:
½ cup dairy or soy milk
¼ teaspoon black tea (optional)

Heat almost to a boil, then pour and serve. You may sweeten the tea with 1 teaspoon honey if desired.

According to yoga nutritional therapy masters, the black pepper is a blood purifier and the cardamom is for the colon, the cloves for the nervous system, and the cinnamon for the bones. Ginger is good for digestion, controlling inflammation, or when you have a cold, the flu, or physical weakness. The milk aids in the easy assimilation of the spices and avoids irritation to the colon and stomach, and the black tea acts as an alloy for all of the ingredients, achieving a new chemical structure, which makes this tea a healthful and delicious drink.

If preparing the tea appears too challenging for you, Yogi Tea may be obtained at your health food store, as well as many traditional supermarkets, either in tea bags or premixed in small cartons.

Dessert: Apple Crumble
Makes 6 servings

5 medium apples, peeled and sliced thin
⅓ cup honey
juice of ½ lemon (about 2 tablespoons)
1 teaspoon grated lemon rind
½ teaspoon cinnamon
⅛ teaspoon nutmeg
1 tablespoon melted butter or ghee
1 cup granola
1 cup apple juice
Optional: ½ cup raisins, ¼ cup mixed nuts, chopped

Place the apples, honey, lemon juice and rind, cinnamon, and nutmeg in a mixing bowl, and stir to combine. Spread in an 8-inch baking dish. In a separate bowl, combine butter and granola and spread over apples, then add the apple juice to provide moisture for cooking. Bake at 350°F for 40 minutes.

May be served with ½ cup nonfat vanilla yogurt per person.

CHAPTER 15

Basic Yoga Nutritional Therapy Recipes

The yoga nutritional therapy program is abundant in life energy. Many of the following foods and recipes have been time-tested for thousands of years.

HEALING DRINKS

According to yoga nutritional therapy, it is best to drink an hour before or after eating, but not during a meal. This allows the digestive enzymes in the stomach to process the food without being diluted by liquids.

In all the following recipes, dairy alternative milks may be used in place of dairy.

Banana Ice Cream or Milk Shake
Makes 1 serving

Bananas are one of nature's perfect foods. This recipe uses frozen bananas. You can keep bananas that are becoming ripe by freezing them with or without peels. If you freeze them with peels, when you are ready to use them, simply run hot water over the bananas, and the skins will come off easily. I recommend keeping the strings underneath the peel because they are rich in minerals.

Place in a blender:
2 frozen bananas, broken into pieces
½ to ⅔ cup milk

Blend all ingredients together until creamy. For ice cream, you may add chopped walnuts, pecans, or carob chips, if desired. For milk shake, add up to 1½ cups milk.

Cardamom-Fennel Tea
Makes 2½ to 3 cups

Both cardamom and fennel promote good digestion, so the combination of the two is especially helpful.

4 cups water
5 crushed open black cardamom pods
or
10 crushed open green cardamom pods (from Asian stores)
1 tablespoon fennel seeds

Boil all ingredients together, then cover and continue boiling for 20 minutes to ½ hour, until the water turns brown. You may need to add approximately ½ cup of water. Add a small amount of milk and honey to taste.

Ginger Tea
Makes 1 serving

Ginger tea is both calming to the nerves and energizing to the body and mind. Although anyone can benefit from drinking ginger tea, this delicious beverage is especially indicated for women during menstruation.

2 cups water
4 to 6 ⅛-inch-thick slices of fresh gingerroot, unpeeled
1 teaspoon lemon juice
1 teaspoon honey

Optional: low-fat milk may be used instead of lemon juice.
Bring water to a boil, and add gingerroot slices. Boil until the water is light brown, about 15 minutes. Add fresh lemon juice and honey.

Golden Milk
Makes 1 to 1½ cups

Turmeric, a root that is ground into a bright yellow powder, is one of the main ingredients in curry. Turmeric is a known anti-inflammatory and is often prescribed in the treatment of many illnesses. It is best known as a lubricant for the joints. It is also excellent for the skin and for the mucous membranes, especially the female reproductive organs. It should always be cooked for at least 5 minutes in water or oil before using. Batches of the cooked solution can be stored in the refrigerator for up to one month, and taken out for use in recipes such as golden milk. To prepare it, simply cook 2 teaspoons of turmeric in 2 cups of pure water for 8 minutes, then let it cool off.

Golden milk is beneficial for the joints, helps relieve pain, and helps to break up calcium deposits that cause stiffness.

¼ to ½ teaspoon turmeric
½ cup water
8 ounces milk
1 tablespoon edible cold-pressed almond oil
1 to 1½ teaspoons honey

Boil turmeric in water for about 8 minutes. You may have to add as much as ½ cup of water. Add milk and almond oil, bring to a boil, then remove from heat and add honey.

Jalapeno Milk
Makes 1 serving

At the first sign of a cold or flu, jalapeno milk is the remedy to stave off sickness because of its high content of vitamin C. Be careful—it is hot! Tip: it is helpful to use frozen jalapenos. When frozen, they are easier to chop, their odor is less harsh, and the juice does not get on the fingers. You can keep frozen jalapenos in a plastic bag in the freezer.

Up to 5 fresh or frozen jalapeno chilies
8 ounces low-fat milk

Blend ingredients together, and sip through a straw. You can start with as little as half a jalapeno pepper and gradually increase the quantity.

Mango Lassi
Makes approximately 4 cups

A lassi (lussee) is a yogurt-based drink. It is great for breakfast or for a snack. Mangoes have been used for ages as a remedy for liver disorders, menstrual problems, and general digestive problems. In combination with fresh yogurt, which contains beneficial bacteria, a mango lassi is a tonic for the entire digestive tract. The combination of mangoes and dairy is a practical example of how foods can balance each other to bring perfect nutrition.

2 cups plain low-fat yogurt
2 medium mangoes, very ripe, peeled and sliced
2 to 3 teaspoons maple syrup or honey
½ cup ice, or ⅔ cup water

Optional: ⅛ teaspoon rosewater (from Asian stores)
Blend all ingredients until smooth and creamy. You may need to add as much as ⅓ cup pure water if the mixture becomes too thick.

Sesame-Ginger Milk
Makes approximately 2 cups

This drink is nourishing to the nervous system and is especially healthful for the male sexual organs, stimulating the production of healthy sexual fluids.

¼ cup sesame seeds
2 tablespoons chopped fresh gingerroot
12 ounces milk
2 teaspoons honey or maple syrup

Blend at high speed until smooth.

Weight-Loss Tea
Makes 2½ to 3 quarts

This tea has been used for centuries to dissolve fatty tissue. Weight-loss tea also improves the beauty and youthfulness of the skin, cleanses the mucous membrane of the colon, and is an excellent source of vitamin C. This tea is a diuretic and helps reduce water retention (which makes up a large part of unwanted weight), balances the appetite, and minimizes food cravings. Drink 2 to 3 glasses per day for weight loss purposes.

Black salt is considered to be a very healing food for cancer prevention. Because it has a strong taste and strong smell, only a very small quantity is used. Tamarind, a sweet and sour tropical fruit, is sold as a paste with or without the seeds.

¼ to ⅓ cup fresh or dried mint leaves
2 cups cumin seeds
1 tablespoon fresh or concentrated tamarind (from Asian stores)
¼ teaspoon black salt (from Asian stores)
4 lemons, sliced
½ tablespoon black pepper
3 quarts water

Combine all the ingredients in a pot and bring to a boil. Lower the heat and continue to boil covered under low heat for two hours. You may have to add as much as ½ quart more water. Strain and serve hot or cold. You can reuse the ingredients to make more tea; just add fresh lemons. This tea can be stored for up to a week in the refrigerator.

ANCIENT YOGA NUTRITIONAL THERAPY RECIPES

ALMONDS

Almonds are an excellent source of protein and a good source of manganese, phosphorus, and potassium. Almond oil is also beneficial both internally and externally for the skin.

In yoga nutritional therapy, it is preferable to eat peeled almonds because the skin is considered to be very astringent. To blanch almonds, soak raw almonds in pure water overnight. Strain the almonds, pour warm water over them, then peel them. You can store unused almonds refrigerated, in a container with enough water to cover them.

ALMOND OIL

Two tablespoons of edible almond oil each day, taken in food or in a smoothie, will help lower cholesterol, reduce body fat and hunger, cleanse the body of toxins, and keep the skin healthy and lustrous. You can use it as salad dressing, in soups, or on grains. You can find almond oil at your local health food store.

BASMATI RICE

This naturally white rice is revered throughout Asia as a sacred food. Basmati is a fragrant, high-quality rice that is not milled or polished, which can strip away most of the vitamin and mineral content of rice. Basmati rice is abundant in B vitamins, iodine, and high-quality protein, and it is easily assimilated. Brown rice, although rich in vitamins, can be hard to digest unless cooked for a very long time in a 4-to-1 ratio with water. White basmati rice cooks in a 2-to-1 ratio with water in about 20 minutes. Rinse two or three times before cooking, then place in cold water. Bring to a boil, then turn to low heat until all water is absorbed and rice is soft.

BEETS

Beets cleanse the liver and digestive tract. They also aid in treating hemorrhoids, eliminating toxins from the body, and regulating blood sugar. To help your body do its own inner cleaning, eat beets every day for one week in the spring or fall.

To prepare beets, cut ½ inch off the greens and steam until soft. Once the beets are soft, run cold water over them as you rub them in your hands. The peels will slide off. Cooked beets can be stored for at least 1 week in the refrigerator. The greens can be lightly steamed or used raw in salads.

If you choose to juice your beets, remember that beet juice is best taken in a 1-to-4 dilution ratio with other juices, such as apple or carrot.

Beet and Carrots Melt
Makes 6 servings

3 green onions, finely chopped
2 teaspoons extra virgin olive oil
½ teaspoon garlic, minced
⅛ teaspoon sea salt
⅛ teaspoon pepper
5 medium beets, cooked, peeled, and grated
6 carrots, steamed, peeled, and grated
⅓ cup grated mild cheese (dairy or nondairy)

Sauté onions in olive oil over medium heat for 5 minutes. Add garlic, sea salt, and pepper, and continue cooking for 5 additional minutes. Add grated beets and carrots, and toss lightly. Sprinkle cheese on top, turn heat to low, and simmer until cheese is melted.

GHEE

In yoga nutritional therapy, ghee is highly regarded as both a nutrient and a preservative for food and medicine. It is also known as clarified butter, because the impurities have been removed through the heating process. Stored in a sealed container, ghee will keep three to four months without refrigeration in mild temperatures. If in doubt, keep refrigerated. It is low in cholesterol and contains no salt.

In a pot, simmer unsalted butter over medium low heat for 10 to 20 minutes, until an almost transparent crust forms on top. Skim off the crust and strain the golden liquid that remains into a container. Make sure to discard the white sediment at the bottom.

Jalapeno Pancakes
Makes 4 medium-small pancakes

In yoga nutritional therapy, jalapeno pancakes are known for their healing properties for colds and the flu. This recipe has been adapted to Western tastes by substituting whole wheat pastry flour for part of the besan flour and by reducing the spices from the original recipe.

½ cup besan (chickpea flour from Asian stores)
⅓ cup whole wheat pastry flour

1 cup milk
¼ teaspoon baking powder
1 teaspoon finely minced or grated ginger
1 clove garlic, finely minced
½ teaspoon coriander seed powder
½ teaspoon sea salt
¼ teaspoon cracked red chilies
½ teaspoon oregano seed
¼ teaspoon black pepper
½ teaspoon cumin seed
1 teaspoon finely chopped jalapeno
10 blanched almonds, finely chopped
2 teaspoons extra virgin olive oil
1 to 2 tablespoons plain low-fat yogurt per person

In a mixing bowl, combine besan and whole wheat pastry flour, then add milk and baking powder—it will make a good pancake consistency. Add remaining ingredients up to and including the almonds. In skillet, heat ⅓ teaspoon or less olive oil per pancake. Place ¼ cup batter, and spread evenly in a circle. Cook until brown on both sides. Serve with yogurt to help digestion and cut the hot, spicy quality of jalapeno.

Masala

The word *masala* means "blend," and this masala is a yogic blend of spices and the trinity roots.

1 tablespoon turmeric
3 teaspoons extra virgin olive oil
2 tablespoons peeled and finely grated ginger
3 cloves garlic, minced
1 yellow onion, chopped

For basic masala, sauté turmeric in olive oil for 5 minutes, then add ginger and cook for 5 minutes. Add garlic and onion. If the mixture starts sticking to the pan, just add a little water. Sauté until all is soft and blended, about 10 minutes. This spice blend will add flavor to vegetables, beans, or grains. Simply mix 1 teaspoon per person into your favorite recipe at the end stage of cooking. Masala may be kept refrigerated for up to 2 weeks. It also freezes perfectly for up to 2 months.

Natural Salad
Makes 6 servings

This is a unique salad that contains no lettuce but is very pleasing to the palate. Fresh parsley adds minerals that cleanse the kidneys and regulate the calcium balance in the body. Parsley has also been shown to be helpful in treating diabetes. Kelp, a dried seaweed, is high in minerals and iodine, which is beneficial to the health of the thyroid gland. Celery aids the nerves, and sunflower seeds add high-quality protein.

1 cup carrots, finely grated
½ cup mild cheese or soy cheese, grated
1 cups breadcrumbs (or small bread cubes)
½ cup raw sunflower seeds
1 cup celery, finely chopped
1 cup parsley, finely chopped
¼ to ½ onion, finely chopped

DRESSING:
1½ tablespoons cold-pressed sesame seed oil or edible almond
    oil
1 to 2 tablespoons Braggs Liquid Aminos or soy sauce
3 tablespoons apple juice
3 tablespoons lemon juice
2 teaspoons basil
1 teaspoon sage
1 teaspoon kelp
3 tablespoons pure water

Place salad ingredients in a bowl. Blend all dressing ingredients together, then toss the salad with the dressing and serve.

Potent Potatoes
Makes 8 servings

4 Russet baking potatoes
2 teaspoons extra virgin olive oil
3 medium onions, chopped
3 tablespoons ginger, minced
2 teaspoons garlic, minced
1 teaspoon crushed red chilies or cayenne pepper (more or
    less to taste)
½ teaspoon ground cloves
1 teaspoon cardamom powder or seeds, or 3 cardamom pods
½ teaspoon ground cinnamon
⅓ cup tamari (soy) sauce
½ pint nonfat cottage cheese

Bake potatoes at 400°F until soft on the inside and crispy on
the outside, approximately 45 minutes. Meanwhile, heat the olive
oil in a skillet, and add onions. Sauté for approximately 10 minutes,
then add ginger and cook for another 5 minutes or until well done,
then add garlic and spices. Add as much as ½ cup pure water if the
mixture sticks. Cook until ingredients all melt together. Add
tamari. Turn off heat. Cut potatoes in half lengthwise when cool
enough to handle. Scoop out insides, leaving enough potato in the
shell so that it does not tear. Combine potato insides with onion
mixture, and add cottage cheese. Refill shells, forming mounds on
top, and serve warm.

Ratatouille
Makes 6 servings

This is considered to be a very healing recipe. Eggplant is considered to be the most powerful food for women, energizing and soothing, and zucchini is excellent for elimination and healthy skin.

1 medium eggplant, peeled, or 8 small Asian eggplants, un-
    peeled
3 medium zucchini
1 onion, finely chopped

2 teaspoons extra virgin olive oil
½ tablespoon each garlic, basil, oregano, dill
½ teaspoon black pepper
1 cup diced tomatoes (fresh or canned)
sea salt or Braggs Liquid Aminos to taste

If using regular-sized eggplant, cut into finger-sized sticks and steam for 5 to 8 minutes. Remove any large clusters of seeds after steaming. If using Asian eggplant, slice in thin rounds and do not steam. Quarter zucchini lengthwise, and cut into 2-inch sticks. Sauté onion in olive oil for 2 minutes, then add garlic and spices, and cook a few minutes more. Add tomatoes, eggplant, and zucchini. Cook until vegetables are soft. Serve with couscous or basmati rice.

Soup of Life
Makes 10 servings

Onions, garlic, and ginger are the three roots of life. Onions invigorate your immune system, garlic has phytonutrients that lower cholesterol, and ginger is a natural anti-inflammatory and digestive tonic. Basil, pepper, and oregano are the three herbs of life. Basil is for the stomach, pepper is for the blood, and oregano seed is known for its healing properties and as a disease preventive. The broth of this soup is very invigorating and keeps well, becoming tastier in the next few days after it is made.

2 teaspoons extra virgin olive oil
2 to 3 yellow onions, sliced thin
¼ cup minced gingerroot
2 teaspoons turmeric
1 teaspoon black pepper
1 tablespoon caraway seeds
½ teaspoon oregano seeds (from Asian stores)
1 tablespoon poppy seeds
1 tablespoon celery seeds
1 tablespoon garam masala
2 to 3 ripe tomatoes, steamed, peeled, and chopped
3 tablespoons basil

1 tablespoon dill weed
1 tablespoon oregano
1 tablespoon tarragon
3 quarts pure water
1 to 2 diced potatoes, unpeeled
2 to 3 carrots, diced
4 cups chopped assorted vegetables
4 tablespoons Braggs Liquid Aminos
3 to 5 cloves garlic, minced

In the bottom of a soup pot, heat the olive oil on medium high heat. Add onions and ginger. If it starts to stick, add a little water. Make a pool in the center of the onion and ginger mixture, then add turmeric, black pepper, caraway seeds, oregano seeds, poppy seeds, celery seeds, and garam masala. Sauté for 2 minutes, then mix well with onions. Add tomatoes and herbs. Add water, potatoes, carrots, and assorted vegetables. Bring to a boil, then simmer over medium heat for about 1 hour. Add Braggs Liquid Aminos and garlic, and simmer 5 minutes longer.

Health-Giving Tofu

It is best to rinse tofu before using and to keep any remaining pieces covered in water in the refrigerator. To minimize the gas-producing quality of tofu, you should not eat it raw. As a rule, use firm tofu for slicing and dicing, and soft tofu for blending.

Baked Tofu
See page 241.

Marinated Tofu
Makes 4 servings

1 package firm tofu (about 16 ounces)
2 teaspoons extra virgin olive oil
¼ cup soy sauce or Braggs Liquid Aminos
1 tablespoon peeled and finely grated ginger
1 clove garlic, finely minced

juice of 1 lemon
¼ cup pure water

Rinse and slice tofu in ½-inch slices. Combine olive oil, soy sauce, ginger, garlic, and lemon juice in the bottom of a glass baking pan. Add the tofu, and let marinate for 2 to 3 hours. Flip tofu once while marinating. Bake at 350°F for 30 minutes. If the marinade evaporates completely and tofu starts sticking, simply add a little water. Serve with sautéed or steamed vegetables.

Tofu Salad
Makes 4 servings

1 package firm tofu (about 16 ounces)
juice of 1 lemon
3 celery sticks, finely diced
⅔ cup grated radishes, carrots, and/or raw zucchini
½ sweet red pepper, finely chopped
2 to 3 dill pickles, finely chopped

DRESSING:
¼ to ½ cup eggless, sugarless mayonnaise (from natural food stores)
2 to 3 tablespoons prepared mustard
1 teaspoon lemon juice
½ teaspoon sea salt
½ teaspoon black pepper

Rinse the tofu and slice it approximately ½ inch thick. Lightly sprinkle with lemon juice, and bake in a lightly oiled baking dish at 375°F until medium hard, about 20 to 25 minutes. Let cool, then grate it.

Meanwhile, in a mixing bowl combine celery, radishes, carrots, zucchini, red pepper, and pickles. Add the grated tofu to the rest of ingredients and mix well. The texture of the grated baked tofu in this dish is similar to that of chicken or tuna salad.

In a small bowl, mix all dressing ingredients and add to the salad. Serve with crackers or with lettuce on bread.

Tofu Spread
Makes approximately 2½ cups

Both tofu and sesame seeds are high in calcium and protein, and both are used in this dish. Tahini is sesame seed paste and can be found at supermarkets, natural food stores, and Middle Eastern stores. Nutritional yeast flakes have a cheesy taste, are high in B vitamins, and are found at natural food stores.

1 pound firm tofu, rinsed and squeezed of excess water
1 to 2 sticks celery, finely diced
1 scallion, finely chopped
⅛ cup fresh parsley, finely chopped
⅛ cup diced sweet red pepper or finely grated carrots

DRESSING:
1 tablespoon lemon juice
⅓ to ½ cup eggless, sugarless mayonnaise
1½ tablespoons nutritional yeast flakes
½ to 1 teaspoon sea salt
1 teaspoon vegetable seasoning such as Jensen's or Spike
2 tablespoons sesame tahini paste

Steam tofu for 5 to 10 minutes. Squeeze any remaining water from the tofu once again. Crumble tofu and mash with the above ingredients. In a separate bowl, mix all dressing ingredients.

Combine tofu mixture with dressing. Serve with crackers or vegetable sticks, or as a sandwich spread.

Wheatberries

The whole wheat "berry," from which wheat flour is milled, is an excellent food when boiled until tender. It cleans the intestinal tract, strengthens the teeth and gums, beautifies the skin, and can help prevent stomach disorders, including cancer.

½ cup wheatberries
5 cups pure water

Soak wheatberries overnight in 2 cups purified water. Drain and cook on medium high heat in 2½ to 3 cups water. Cook until the wheat is puffed up and tender, about 1 hour. Wheatberries can also be cooked overnight in a crock pot.

Wheatberries are delicious as a breakfast cereal blended with milk and honey, or as a main dish with masala.

Yogurt Curry
Makes 4 servings

Yogurt curry soothes and strengthens the nervous system and pleases the palate.

    3 cups chopped mixed vegetables, such as broccoli, carrots,
        cauliflower, and peas
    1 cup white basmati rice
    1 cup low-fat yogurt
    ¼ cup besan (chickpea flour from Asian stores)
    1 cup pure water
    1 tablespoon turmeric
    ¼ teaspoon oregano seeds
    ¼ teaspoon cumin seeds
    ¼ teaspoon ground black pepper
    1 teaspoon garam masala
    3 teaspoons ghee
    2 small onions, finely chopped
    2 cloves garlic, minced
    ¼ cup minced ginger

Steam chopped mixed vegetables until tender and set them aside. Make basmati rice according to recipe on page 145 and set aside. Blend yogurt and besan flour with 1 cup of water until smooth, and set the mixture aside. Sauté turmeric, oregano and cumin seeds, black pepper, and garam masala in ghee until golden brown. Add chopped onion, garlic, and ginger. Simmer until mixture is blended, about 5 minutes. Stir in yogurt-flour mixture. Simmer until sauce thickens. Serve over rice and steamed vegetables.

PART 2

Eat This for That

CHAPTER 16

Addictions

Addiction is one of the greatest maladies facing the world today. In my experience, addictions are a form of self-medication, a substitute for missing vitamins, minerals, or trace elements. Yoga nutritional therapy, as part of an integrated medical program that includes meditation, acupuncture, and massage, has proved to be very successful in eliminating problems with drugs, alcohol, and nicotine.

DIET

To combat addictions, the basic yoga nutritional therapy diet should be followed (see page 128). Also, following a monodiet of mung beans and rice for seven days (see page 80) is especially cleansing and nurturing.

Drug addiction is obviously a very difficult problem. This dietary program, while challenging, has stood the test of time. It has been effective even in the hardest cases, including heroin addiction.

Other therapies to be used in conjunction with this program are acupuncture and therapeutic massage. In addition, here are a few specific food prescriptions for alleviating the symptoms of addiction:

- For extreme restlessness, massage the feet with a mixture of garlic juice and almond oil. Garlic improves respiration and lowers blood pressure, and its juice is readily absorbed through all the nerves that end in the feet, having a positive effect on all the internal organs and the brain.

- To help wake up after using sedatives or alcohol, drink mint tea and garlic juice, immediately after practicing a simple breathing technique, Sitali Pranayama, for 10 minutes. Breathe in through the mouth, with the tongue rolled up lengthwise and slightly sticking out of the mouth. Then breathe out through the nose. Garlic juice is an excellent blood purifier, helping to eliminate excess alcohol from the system. Mint tea accelerates detoxification and improves digestion.

- To increase energy, drink pineapple juice (canned juice is okay). This juice provides pure, easily assimilable energy to the body via its natural sweetness.

- While you are quitting cigarettes, eat one pack of raisins a day. Raisins are very rich in antioxidants and minerals, and they effectively replace the habit of smoking cigarettes.

SUPPLEMENTS AND SPECIFIC NUTRIENTS

Primary

Everyone should take a high-potency multiple vitamin and mineral supplement, as explained in the fifth principle (see page 120). In addition, to support the body during active addictions and during withdrawal, the following nutrients are recommended:

Vitamin C: Take 3,000 to 9,000 mg per day in three divided doses. Alcohol and smoking cause depletion of vitamin C; therefore, taking it will help restore the amount of the vitamin in the body.

Secondary

Coenzyme Q10: 100 to 300 mg per day will aid in the generation of cellular energy.

HERBS

Primary

Ginseng: 75 to 150 mg panax ginseng and 150 to 300 mg Siberian ginseng per day will help detoxify and normalize the functioning of the entire system.

Milk thistle: 320 mg per day, with meals. Use solid extract with 80 percent silymarin. Milk thistle protects against toxins and pollutants, and it promotes the production of liver cells.

Secondary
Kava kava: 150 mg up to six times per day for anxiety. Check with your health care practitioner concerning potential liver problems. Kava kava also helps with insomnia and stress-related disorders.

St. John's wort: 300 mg 3 times per day for depression. St. John's wort additionally helps control stress and is a natural mood booster.

JUICES

The following seven-day juicing regimen has been successful in alleviating addictions at The SuperHealth Ranch, where I was medical director. These juices are very effective in detoxifying the body and providing key nutrition to rejuvenate the blood and the internal organs. You can follow this regimen in the comfort of your home, in addition to your meals. Only organic fruits and vegetables should be used.

To prepare the juices, wash and dry all ingredients. Peel cucumbers and pineapple before juicing.

7:00 A.M.	1 cup warm water, 1 tablespoon lemon juice, 1 teaspoon rosewater
	Alternate every other day with 1 cup orange juice, ½ tablespoon ginger juice
10:00 A.M.	½ cup fresh cucumber juice, ½ cup fresh celery juice
3:00 P.M.	
Sunday	⅓ cup fresh beet juice, ⅓ cup fresh carrot juice, ⅓ cup fresh pineapple juice
Monday	⅓ cup fresh beet juice, ⅓ cup fresh carrot juice, ⅓ cup fresh pineapple juice
Tuesday	½ cup fresh apple juice, ½ cup fresh celery juice
Wednesday	⅓ cup fresh beet juice, ⅓ cup fresh carrot juice, ⅓ cup fresh pineapple juice
Thursday	⅓ cup fresh grape juice, ⅓ cup fresh apple juice, ⅓ cup fresh carrot juice
Friday	½ cup fresh apple juice, ½ cup fresh celery juice
Saturday	⅓ cup fresh grape juice, ⅓ cup fresh apple juice, ⅓ cup fresh celery juice

The lemon with water, taken first thing in the morning, has a very calming effect on the digestive system, aiding elimination and burning fat. Orange and ginger juices are powerful antioxidants and anti-inflammatory agents. Cucumber and celery juices are very soothing to the nervous system and provide high amounts of crucial minerals for optimal health. Beet-carrot-pineapple juice stimulates the digestive system and the liver, and normalizes the entire system. Apple-celery juice flushes the kidneys, helps the digestive system, nourishes the muscles, and relieves stress. Grape-apple-carrot juice normalizes the system, accelerates metabolism, and facilitates the expulsion of toxins from the body. Grape-apple-celery juice is relaxing to the nervous system, boosts the immune system, and enhances the digestive function.

RECIPE

A traditional yoga nutritional therapy recipe for breaking addictions is a banana fast. Here's how to do it.

Breakfast

Drink 1 cup of freshly squeezed orange juice, with the pulp, sweetened with 1 teaspoon of honey. After 1 hour, eat three bananas, making sure you eat the strings inside the peel. Chew thoroughly, until each bite is liquid, before you swallow it. Immediately after the bananas, chew the seeds of one cardamom pod.

Lunch

Three bananas, followed by the seeds of one cardamom pod.

Dinner

Three bananas, followed by the seeds of one cardamom pod.

Remember to drink at least eight glasses of room-temperature water per day. You may also drink Yogi Tea or another herbal tea.

The banana fast is not recommended for people who have not followed a fast before. If you have never fasted, follow the mung beans and rice diet for seven days before trying the banana fast. As with any fast, you may feel weak, emotional, or short-tempered at the beginning. These symptoms will gradually go away. If constipation becomes a problem, gradually increase the cardamom up to three pods after each meal.

This fast removes drug deposits from the medulla in the brain. I recommend beginning on the day of the new moon and continuing for fourteen days, until the full moon. It will work on building up worn tissues and adjusting the iron, sodium, and potassium balance in the body.

To break the fast
On the fifteenth day, drink only warm water with a little lemon juice and honey. Then start a monodiet of mung beans and rice (see page 80) for twenty-eight days. Yogi Tea can also be used. Follow the basic mung beans and rice recipe on page 80, with the following modifications:

- Instead of 1 cup of mung beans and 1 of rice, use ½ cup of each.
- Together with the spices, add some fresh or dried mint leaves.

At the end of the twenty-eight days, gradually add salads and fruit. Use dairy and wheat last.

CHAPTER 17

Allergies

Allergies are increasing in the population because of greater exposure to environmental pollutants and food contamination. However, dietary modification, vitamins, nutrients, and herbs can play a major role in reducing allergic reactions.

If you have allergies, the most important thing to do is to detoxify your body with a short fast, as described in the first principle (see page 70). Then make sure you go organic, and be very careful not to eat any GMO foods. Use plant sources, rather than animal products, as the main source of protein in your diet. Another worthwhile practice is to remove all dairy products from your diet.

If your allergies remain severe after your short fast, you must be extra mindful of your diet. Keep a food log for a week and then repeat your short fast, slowly adding one food at a time. In this way you can discover which foods induce an allergic reaction. The most common foods causing allergy are eggs, wheat, white potatoes, dairy, soy, peanuts, and sometimes oranges.

DIET

You may have to look no further than the mung beans and rice recipe to solve your allergy problems (see page 80). This particular food combination and the way it is prepared provide good nutrition while gently eliminating toxins and easing the demands on your digestive system. Many people have cleansed their system by following this as a monodiet for a week or more. You can vary the taste by adding salsa or other spices. If things are going well—that is, there is a reduction in symptoms—then add salmon for its source of omega-3s to reduce inflammatory signals sent to your immune system. Of course, eating an abundance of green leafy vegetables with their wide array of phytonutrients and antioxidants will help saturate your system and reduce the contribution of free radicals to the allergic response.

Because people with allergies are usually deficient in manganese, the diet should be varied to add buckwheat, beans, peas, and blueberries, which are all rich in this nutrient.

SUPPLEMENTS AND SPECIFIC NUTRIENTS

Primary

Everyone should take a high-potency multiple vitamin and mineral supplement, as explained in the fifth principle (see page 120). In addition, to prevent allergies I recommend taking the following nutrients daily:

Bioflavonoids: A good way to obtain bioflavonoids is to take 100 mg of grapeseed extract three times a day. Bioflavonoids work synergistically with vitamin C.

Coenzyme Q10: Take 100 mg per day. Coenzyme Q10 improves immune function.

Vitamin C: Take up to 12,000 mg in six divided doses per day. If you develop stomach upset or diarrhea, simply reduce the dose. Vitamin C aids in the production of antistress hormones and in the production of immune system proteins.

Secondary

DHEA: In addition to its strong anti-aging properties, DHEA has significant anti-allergy properties. If you are not already taking it as part of your anti-aging program, DHEA may be taken at a dose of 25 to 100 mg per day to decrease allergy symptoms.

Remember to have your DHEA blood level measured by your doctor before adding it to your daily supplements. Also, men must have a prostate-specific antigen (PSA) test, and in most cases a prostate examination by the doctor, before adding this supplement to their daily diet. Men will then need to repeat the DHEA blood level and PSA tests every six months. Women, of course, will need to repeat only their DHEA test every six months. For more information on DHEA, see page 169.

Magnesium: Additional magnesium at a dose of 500 to 1,000 mg per day is particularly helpful if your allergies are causing asthmalike symptoms. Magnesium helps with stress reduction and alleviates anxiety, tension, and muscular spasms.

N-acetylcysteine: Good antiallergic results have been obtained with the powerful antioxidant *N*-acetylcysteine. I recommend up to 600 mg per day. *N*-acetylcysteine is a powerful detoxifier of substances such as alcohol and other toxins, which can cause suppression of the immune system.

Omega-3 oil: Take 1,500 mg per day. An omega-3 supplement in the form of gamma-linolenic acid from borage oil helps control allergies.

Pantothenic acid: If stress is a contributing factor to your allergies, then you may add extra B vitamins to your multiple vitamin, especially 300 to 500 mg of pantothenic acid (vitamin B_5). It tones both the adrenal glands and the thymus, which are crucial in the fight against allergies.

HERBS
Primary
Stinging nettle: Take 750 mg per day. Stinging nettle is good for the immune system and has been reported to aid in treating severe allergies.

JUICE
Antiallergy Smoothie
Makes 1 serving

2 slices cantaloupe, peeled
¼ inch gingerroot, peeled
½ apple

Optional
¼ scoop of Longevity Green Drink (see Appendix E, Resources) or other green powder

Wash and dry all the ingredients, then juice them. Fresh juices are best consumed within 2 or 3 hours of preparation and should be refrigerated.

Cantaloupe, ginger, and apple boost the immune system, detoxify the gastrointestinal tract, and soothe the digestive system. This rejuvenates the internal organs, which helps to alleviate allergy symptoms.

RECIPE

Please see the mung beans and rice recipe on page 80.

CHAPTER 18

Anti-Aging

I was one of the thirteen original doctors and scientists of the American Academy of Anti-Aging Medicine (A4M). At our first meeting in Chicago in 1991, we discussed the formation of a professional organization that would have as its mission the extension of health and life span. Since then, anti-aging medicine has grown exponentially. Today the A4M counts over 5,000 committed individuals as members. We have learned a lot since 1991, and I will share some accumulated knowledge with you in the following pages. If you take my advice, you will soon notice an improvement in your physical, mental, emotional, and spiritual well-being. You will also add productive and enjoyable years to your life.

The fountain of youth that we all seek is inside us. We only have to activate it. While every idea, principle, and recipe in this book will prolong your life and make your years more enjoyable, there are a few particular dietary and nutrient supplementation tips that will help you to specifically activate your longevity genes and turn off your aging ones. Also, the modern concept of artful hormone replacement therapy plays a significant role in living an enhanced life. Anti-aging has really become age management.

DIET

First, you must follow all seven principles outlined in this book. Next, you must eat a diet reasonably low in saturated fats that includes seeds, nuts, grains, beans, high-quality protein such as fish, and especially soy foods. Try to make the transition to a completely plant-based diet if you so desire, but at the very least, limit your consumption of animal protein, especially red meat, to no more than twice a week. Also, reduce your consumption of eggs to four a week, and eliminate all fried foods. Avoid processed foods such as white bread, white flour, and fast foods, but do remember to have your seven to nine servings of fresh organic fruit and vegetables each and every day—especially broccoli sprouts, cabbage, cauliflower, tomatoes, blueberries, and apples.

As you age you should decrease your overall calorie consumption and increase the amount of raw foods you eat. Make sure you drink eight glasses of pure (bottled or filtered) water per day. Add plenty of garlic, onions, ginger, and chilies to your diet, as your taste and digestion permit, because of their rich array of age-fighting nutrients. Limit your alcohol consumption to an occasional glass of red wine, and reduce the salt in your diet.

SUPPLEMENTS AND SPECIFIC NUTRIENTS

Primary

Everyone should take a high-potency vitamin and mineral supplement as described in the fifth principle (see page 120). In addition, to combat the negative effects of aging, I suggest taking the following specific nutrients:

Coenzyme Q10: 100 to 300 mg per day. Coenzyme Q10 plays an important role in the production of energy in all cells of the body, stimulates the immune system, and has very important anti-aging effects.

Alpha-lipoic acid: 250 mg per day. Alpha-lipoic acid is a potent antioxidant, which helps liver function.

Vitamin E: Up to 800 IU per day. Vitamin E inhibits cell damage and the creation of free radicals. It slows down aging and the progression of Alzheimer's disease.

Vitamin C: Up to 10,000 mg per day, as tolerated. Vitamin C promotes the growth and repair of tissue and participates in at least three hundred metabolic processes in the body.

Digestive enzymes: 1 to 2 capsules or tablets with each meal, depending on what supplement you use. Digestive enzymes promote optimal absorption of nutrients in the body.

Green tea: 1 or 2 cups per day, decaffeinated. Green tea contains chemicals that have health-enhancing properties.

Secondary
Indole-3-carbinol: 150 mg three times per day. Indole-3-carbinol is very effective in fighting free radical and DNA damage.

N-Acetylcysteine: Up to 500 mg per day. N-acetylcysteine increases the levels of protective enzymes in the body, thus slowing some of the damage in the cells that is caused by aging.

HERBS
Primary
Ginkgo: 120 mg in the morning. Ginkgo increases blood flow and raises the oxygen supply to all parts of the body, including the heart and the brain.

Secondary
Ginseng: 150 mg per day of panax ginseng and/or 300 mg of Siberian ginseng per day. Too much ginseng may raise your blood pressure. Take care not to exceed the recommended dosage. Ginseng fights against weakness, provides additional energy, and increases longevity.

Astragalus: 500 mg four times per day. Astragalus guards the immune system, aids with adrenal gland function, and promotes healing. No side effects have been reported at this recommended dose.

A BRIEF DISCUSSION OF HORMONE REPLACEMENT THERAPY
"Hormone replacement therapy is a promising strategy."

"No one should go around injecting themselves with anti-aging hormones."

The same physician, who shall remain anonymous, made both of these statements. The first was at a professional meeting I attended, and the second was in an interview for a general magazine. This dichotomy highlights the controversy surrounding the art and science of hormone replacement therapy.

I use hormone replacement therapy in my practice and find it very beneficial. For example, an older man recently came to me because he was literally about to die. He had no energy, his memory was gone, and his diabetes was out of control. He also couldn't breathe because of weakness and underlying lung disease. I measured his hormones and found them to be incredibly low, almost incompatible with life. I replaced the almost nonexistent levels of testosterone and DHEA but could not replace human growth hormone because of its expense. Still, he improved so fast that in a few weeks he was able to travel around the country, visiting relatives he had thought about while preparing to die.

Many doctors who practice anti-aging medicine have had similar experiences using hormone replacement therapy. Those with little experience in this specialty caution against it, saying there is not enough research. I disagree. There is enough supportive clinical work to allow for careful hormone replacement therapy in selected persons. There are important considerations, however:

- Hormone levels in the blood must be measured. If they are low, it makes sense to replace them in an informed manner. If they are not low, it is not safe to boost them higher than normal.
- The hormone levels should be restored to the naturally occurring levels of a thirty-year-old, and never younger.
- Blood tests must be repeated every six months or as needed to monitor hormone levels.

The hormones I measure include DHEA, estrogen, human growth hormone, progesterone, testosterone, and thyroid hormone. Although I, like many physicians in this specialty, don't measure melatonin and pregnenolone, I replace them when that is clinically indicated. I know of no patient treated by anti-aging medicine specialists who has had life-threatening, severe, or uncontrollable side effects from hormone replacement therapy.

Here is a brief description of each important hormone and the symptoms of low levels in your body.

DHEA
I have discussed DHEA on page 117. I use it extensively and have never been disappointed by the results. DHEA protects your heart, stimulates the immune system, restores sexual vitality, improves mood, and has a positive effect on the way your body looks. Perhaps most important, DHEA brings back the "juice of life." As with any other hormone, you should take DHEA under the supervision of your physician.

Please see the chart on page 176 for dosing information.

Estrogen

The ovaries in women secrete estrogen. Estrogen is responsible for keeping the skin youthful looking and moist, enhancing muscle tone, and maintaining natural lubrication of the vaginal mucous membranes. It also maximizes immune function. Reduced levels of estrogen have been related to an increased incidence of Alzheimer's disease, as well as menopause-related symptoms such as hot flashes, osteoporosis, anxiety, and reduced libido.

Premarin, the estrogen replacement drug most often prescribed by conventional doctors, is composed of the urine of pregnant horses. Is that what you want to put in your body? A better choice is one of two natural forms of estrogen: Biest, a mixture of 80 percent estriol and 20 percent estradiol, or Tri-est, a balanced combination of 10 to 20 percent estradiol, 10 to 20 percent estrone, and 60 to 80 percent estriol.

As new information is constantly being discovered about estrogen replacement therapy, you should always discuss the potential harmful effects of estrogen with your doctor.

Please see the chart on page 176 for dosing information.

Human growth hormone (hGH)

If ever there was hope for a fountain of youth in an injection, hGH is it. Since it started making its way into clinical medicine in the early 1990s, hGH has been the subject of books, television shows, and discussions around the world.

Does it really work? Is it dangerous?

What's clear is that the reduced production of hGH in your body with age is at least partially, if not completely, responsible for a significant amount of the general signs of aging. These include

- Decreased energy and fatigue
- Lack of well-being
- Lack of drive and motivation
- Decreased ability and desire to exercise
- Loss of concentration, sociability, and activity
- Decreased sleep
- Poor response to stress
- Memory difficulties
- Irritability and mood disorders

The physical body responds to a loss of hGH with

- Sagging muscles
- Increased abdominal fat
- Decreased muscle strength
- Loose skin
- Wrinkles
- Thinning hair
- Poor posture

Diminished hGH may lead to

- Poor healing
- Increased fat in the blood
- Decreased bone density
- Heart disease from arteriosclerosis
- Decreased immune response
- Poor kidney function
- Possibly cancer

According to research studies by Daniel Rudman, M.D., published in the New England Journal Of Medicine in 1991, as well as a vast amount of clinical experience by Sam Baxas, M.D., Neal Rozier, M.D., David Leonardi, M.D., Ronald Klatz, D.O., the late Leo M. Levin, M.D., and myself, it appears that growth hormone replacement therapy results in

- Decreased body fat
- Increased energy and exercise capacity
- Increased quality of life and vitality
- Increased muscle size and strength, especially if you exercise
- Improved bone growth and strength
- Increased healing, for example after injury or surgery
- Improved sense of well-being
- Better-looking skin, decreased wrinkles
- Improved heart function
- Increased hair, skin, and nail growth
- Improved memory and brain function

- Improved sleep
- Improved lung function and capacity
- Less fat in the blood
- Improved immunity, with possibly less cancer
- Increased life expectancy and quality of life (disease prevention)
- A younger-looking you

So what is the downside?

I don't think there is a downside to hGH replacement therapy if it is practiced wisely. I always measure the lab values of hGH and don't over-replace the hormone. However, I must say that while I know of no long-term side effects when hGH is prescribed and taken in a reasonable manner, all the answers are not yet in. I always suggest following the philosophy of risk/benefit ratio. Let's say that a person who is elderly and suffering is much more concerned about the quality of life now than about the possible side effects later. In my view, why not allow that person to live out his or her life with the highest quality possible? Replacement therapy with hGH does that.

If, on the other hand, you are still relatively young—say in your fifties—but have symptoms of premature aging and are aware that there may be potential risks down the road, you can choose to try it or not. But remember, you can always try it and stop.

hGH therapy is not for men only. One of my greatest therapeutic success stories using hGH was in a woman with a severe form of arthritis. Before hGH replacement therapy, she was bent over, immobile, and in pain. Afterward, she became so strong and pain free that she built a lap pool in her back yard so she could swim every day.

If you or someone you know chooses to take hGH, you will inevitably have more questions. Here are answers to three commonly asked questions about hGH:

1. *What about the cost?* The cost of hGH replacement therapy can be prohibitive for many people, as it may be close to $1,000 per month. Although some patients and doctors take time off from the injections, in general it should be taken for the rest of your life.

2. *What about using oral growth hormone releasing formulas?* These oral products contain a mixture of amino acids thought to release hGH from your own pituitary gland. My professional opinion is that if you need hGH, you should take the real thing. If you absolutely can't afford

it, the oral growth hormone releasing formulas can be tried, but I am not convinced they work to raise the amount of hGH in your body to a therapeutic level.

3. *What about the use of sublingual homeopathic growth hormone?* Again, if you need hGH, I think you should take the real thing. I have not seen conclusive studies that show sublingual homeopathic growth hormone to be clinically effective.

Please see the chart on page 176 for dosing information.

Melatonin

Melatonin is the hormone produced by your pineal gland, one of your master glands in the brain, along with the hypothalamus and the pituitary gland. Although melatonin was originally thought to be only a sleep hormone, we now know that it also plays a role as a key antioxidant in your body. For that reason, melatonin replacement is being studied as a form of cancer therapy.

The amount of melatonin secreted by the pineal gland decreases with age, which creates sleeping difficulties in many of my patients. Therefore, I quite often replace it. I have found that the required dose can vary widely. Some people require only a small dose, say 0.5 mg at bedtime, to get a good night's sleep. Others may need 3 mg or more. The correct dose is the amount that induces sleep rapidly, allows you to sleep through the night (ideally not even getting up to go to the bathroom), and permits you to wake up refreshed in the morning without feeling groggy.

I have found that people who take care of their brains (see page 184) need only a fraction of the dose needed by those who do not follow a brain longevity program.

Please see the chart on page 176 for dosing information.

Pregnenolone

Pregnenolone is the grandmother of all the other hormones. In the biochemistry of the body, it is the one from which all others are formed. That means you must have an adequate amount of pregnenolone for your body to produce DHEA. After pregnenolone helps form DHEA, men and women use it differently. In women, pregnenolone is converted to estrogen; in men, it is converted into testosterone.

Pregnenolone functions as a memory hormone. The brain even has specific receptors for it. Research on pregnenolone was initially done in the 1940s. At that time, two studies demonstrated the effect of pregnenolone on enhancing memory. The first tested the mental skills of pilots and subjects who were not pilots on a flight simulator. Some of the subjects were given pregnenolone, and some were given a placebo. After two weeks of testing, regardless of previous flight training, those who received the hormone did much better with the flight simulator than those in the placebo group.

The second study looked at factory workers who were paid by the piece. The results of the study showed an increase in total productivity, fewer errors, and a better quality of the finished product in those taking pregnenolone, who also reported having more energy, less fatigue, improved mood, and better ability to cope with stress.

Pregnenolone is also helpful in reducing the pain of arthritis, and has a successful treatment history dating back sixty years to prove it. Before the advent of cortisone, which has many undesirable side effects, users of pregnenolone reported less pain and increased mobility from taking pregnenolone tablets.

One of my most gratifying professional experiences concerns the use of pregnenolone. In 1995, I was asked to see a ninety-one-year-old woman with a Ph.D. in psychology. As amazing as it sounds, she was still practicing until she started losing her memory, perhaps a year before her daughter brought her to see me. Unfortunately, she was deteriorating rapidly, and her family feared she might have to go into assisted living.

Pregnenolone came to this woman's rescue. I began by prescribing 100 mg a day, the highest I have ever used, combined with 10 mg a day of the brain longevity medicine deprenyl. Her recovery was dramatic—so much so that my local television station did a program about her. She returned to being a part-time practicing psychologist and an elder in her church.

Please see the chart on page 176 for dosing information.

Progesterone

Progesterone is secreted by the ovary and reduces the symptoms of premenstrual syndrome (PMS). It also decreases the headache and bloating associated with menstruation. Natural progesterone is protective against breast cancer, osteoporosis, fibrocystic disease, and ovarian cysts. It is often a forgotten player in hormone replacement therapy because many doctors treat its ability to enhance quality of life as relatively unimportant. However, replacing low levels of progesterone can make a big difference in a woman's total health and well-being.

Please see the chart on page 176 for dosing information.

Testosterone

Maintaining youthful levels of testosterone is very important for the long-term health and vitality of both men and women. Testosterone is secreted by the ovaries, adrenal glands, and testes. Healthy levels of testosterone in the body result in increased muscle mass, strength, and endurance; decreased fat; increased exercise tolerance; enhancement of well-being; improvement in lean muscle mass; stronger bones; decreased cholesterol; improved skin tone; better healing; increased libido; and heightened sexuality.

Testosterone also prolongs the quality of life by decreasing the diseases of aging. It protects against cardiovascular disease, hypertension, obesity, and arthritis. Replacing testosterone levels when they are low also enhances memory. In fact, there is medical evidence to support the notion that all of the body's systems are rejuvenated by testosterone.

Please see the chart on page 176 for dosing information.

Testosterone for women

Women naturally secrete testosterone from their ovaries. Testosterone is needed in the female body to maintain strong bones, thus preventing osteoporosis. When low levels of this hormone are replaced in menopausal women, their libido returns to normal, and muscle strength and endurance are improved.

Please see the chart on page 176 for dosing information.

Thyroid hormone

Thyroid hormone regulates temperature, metabolism, and brain function. When thyroid hormone is at the proper level in the body, it breaks down fat, helps you lose weight, and lowers your cholesterol. Thyroid hormone also protects against heart disease and cognitive loss, and it relieves sparse hair, dry skin, and thin nails.

As we age, our levels of thyroid hormone decrease. The problem is that many conventional doctors don't treat the problem until the patient has been suffering needlessly for too long. Why? Because they pay too much attention to the laboratory value of the thyroid hormone rather than the patient's symptoms. That's why at my medical training programs I always ask, "Are you going to treat the number or the patient? When I look out at the doctors taking my program, it's as if a light goes on, and they get it. You see, physicians are taught to wait until the lab values are completely abnormal *before* prescribing thyroid hormone. I believe, as do many anti-aging doctors, that a person with a low-normal blood level of the thyroid hormone, but who has symptoms, deserves treatment. And patients are very grateful. In fact, it is well known that doctors receive more bouquets of flowers from patients whose low-normal levels of thyroid have been corrected than from anyone else! The chart below depicts the lab test and hormone replacement doses I recommend.

Hormone chart

Before replacing DHEA, estrogen, hGH, progesterone, testosterone, or thyroid hormones, you must have the hormone levels in the blood measured. Following is a chart of blood tests I recommend to measure hormone levels. It also includes laboratory values and treatment suggestions.

Hormone	Lab values (may vary according to laboratory)	Treatment
DHEA, men	146–850	25–100 mg per day
DHEA, women	112–722	25–100 mg per day
Free testosterone, men	7.2–24	10–50 mg in a cream applied once or twice per day (some doctors use weekly injection)
Free testosterone, women	Premenopausal: 1.1–8.5	2–8 mg in a cream applied once or twice per day
	Postmenopausal: 0.6–6.7	2–8 mg in a cream applied once or twice per day
TSH (marker of thyroid)	0.35–500	½ grain–3 grains per day

Free T3 (thyroid hormone)	2.3–4.2	See TSH
Free T4 (thyroid hormone)	0.70–1.53	See TSH
Estradiol (estrogen) (for women only)	25–443	Bi-Est 2.5–5 mg per day Tri-Est 2.5–5 mg per day
Progesterone (for women only)	150–300	100–300 mg twice per day
hGH (measured as IgF1, also called somatomedin C)	260–350	3–8 units per week by injection under the skin
Melatonin	Not usually measured	0.1–3 mg for sleep; higher doses for cancer therapy (see page 193 for more information)
Pregnenolone	Not usually measured	10–100 mg per day

JUICE

Dr. Dharma's Anti-Aging Cocktail
Makes 1 serving

½ papaya
2 fresh apricots
½ mango
1 cup unsweetened pineapple juice (canned is okay)
½ cup ice
water as needed

Optional
Add ¼ scoop of Longevity Green Drink (see Appendix E, Resources) or other green powder, and/or 1 scoop of non-GMO soy or whey protein powder

Wash and dry papaya, apricots, and mango. Peel and take out the seed from the papaya, peel mango, and take pits from the apricots. Place all ingredients in a blender or Vita-Mix and blend well. Fresh juices are best consumed within 2 or 3 hours of preparation and should be refrigerated.

These fruits contain high amounts of minerals, vitamins, and fiber, which are very beneficial to maintaining healthy skin, circulation to all the internal organs, good vision, and proper digestion.

RECIPES

See mung beans and rice recipe on page 80, or try the rainbow plate recipe.

The Rainbow Plate
Makes 4 servings

4 small beets, peeled and sliced
2 cups broccoli florets
2 cups kale
½ cup edamame soy beans
⅓ onion, chopped
2 teaspoons garlic, minced
1 teaspoon ginger, minced
2 teaspoons extra virgin olive oil
4 veggie burgers

DRESSING:
½ cup low-fat cottage cheese
1 tablespoon tahini paste
1 clove garlic
2 tablespoons lemon juice
2 teaspoons Braggs Liquid Aminos
1 tablespoon parsley
¼ teaspoon sea salt
1 tablespoon pure water

Wash and dry all ingredients. First, put beets in the steamer and cook for 20 minutes or until soft. Add the broccoli, kale, and edamame soy beans. Steam for 5 to 8 more minutes.

In the meantime, sauté onion, garlic, and ginger in olive oil for 3 minutes, or until light brown. Add the veggie burgers and cook for 2 to 3 minutes, then flip them and cook for another 2 to 3 minutes. If pan becomes sticky, add a little water.

In food processor, blend all dressing ingredients until smooth. Serve on individual plates with the veggie burger in the middle and the vegetables arranged all around it. Drizzle 2 tablespoons of dressing per plate on top of the vegetables.

The rainbow plate is an important example of the ideal way of eating. All these vegetables provide antioxidants, phytonutrients, fiber, and trace elements necessary to slow the aging process. Experiment with different vegetables that create a rainbow on your plate.

Ninety percent of the things you can do to prolong your life are related to your lifestyle. After you have your diet—including vitamins, exercise, and stress reduction—in place, it is reasonable to consider hormone replacement therapy, if you are still symptomatic. Having said that, however, I have seen some people with very low hormone levels who didn't have the zest to exercise. For such people, I believe it is permissible to begin hormone replacement therapy and then begin exercising.

CHAPTER 19

Attention Deficit Disorder (ADD) and Attention Deficit Hyperactivity Disorder (ADHD)

Attention deficit disorder afflicts at least 5 percent of school-aged children, with boys being diagnosed ten times more often than girls. The symptoms include a poor attention span, concentration difficulties, and impulsiveness. When hyperactivity is also present, the diagnosis is attention deficit hyperactivity disorder.

Children are not the only ones with these conditions. In fact, I have several patients who have had these symptoms their whole life but were never diagnosed.

Aggravating factors for ADD and ADHD include stress, fatigue, alcohol consumption, and caffeine and sugar intake. Soda pops are loaded with both caffeine and sugar and are thus especially harmful. I once had a patient who brought his young son to see me because of ADHD. I prescribed a change of diet as the first step. A couple of days later, I saw the boy on his way to school, and he was drinking a cola! Obviously, the sugar and caffeine content in the drink were playing a major role in his hyperactivity.

DIET

A diet based on complex carbohydrates, with approximately 30 percent high-quality protein and no more than 20 percent fat, is the ideal diet for both children and adults with this condition. Be sure to incorporate fish into the diet, too. Fish is extremely beneficial for everyone, but especially for those with ADD and ADHD. In addition to the omega-3 fatty acids, fish contains coenzyme Q10, which is important for ideal brain function.

SUPPLEMENTS AND SPECIFIC NUTRIENTS

Primary

Adults should take a high-potency multiple vitamin and mineral supplement, as explained in the fifth principle (see page 120). Special multivitamins for children and adolescents can be found in your local health food store.

In addition, I recommend taking a green product daily, in either pill or powder form. Green products contain plant extracts, which help to increase focus and concentration. Patients report a feeling of waking up their brain, or a lifting of the mental fog, after taking them. This feeling is provided by the trace elements in the green product that are absorbed immediately into the bloodstream and go directly to the brain. Of the many green products on the market, I recommend Longevity Green Drink (see Appendix E, Resources).

Decohexanoic acid (DHA), fish oil, and flaxseed oil are also quite helpful with concentration and brain function, especially in children and adolescents. I once treated a mother and her two teenage daughters who had ADD. In addition to dietary modification, supplementation with DHA brought both girls back to their previous high levels of achievement in school. For proper doses, see the chart below.

Stimulant drugs such as Ritalin are tremendously overused in the treatment of ADD and ADHD. Parents should teach children good eating habits and monitor their diets as much as possible. If you are an adult with ADD or ADHD, you must watch your own diet. With improved diet and proper supplementation, the use of Ritalin will be markedly reduced. Since we don't know the long-term effects of Ritalin and other stimulant medications, the less you use them, the better off you're likely to be.

	Children under 12	Adults
DHA (decohexanoic acid)	10–50 mg/day	500–1,000 mg/day
or		
Fish oil	100 mg/day	500–1,000 mg/day
or		
Flaxseed oil	100 mg/day	500–1,000 mg/day

HERBS

Primary

Ginkgo: Up to 120 mg per day for adults helps with focus. Ginkgo is not recommended for children or adolescents.

JUICE

Fruit Salad Cocktail
Makes 1 serving

1 medium bunch grapes
½ apple
¼ lemon, peeled

Wash and dry ingredients. Juice all the ingredients together. Fresh juices are best consumed within 2 to 3 hours of preparation and should be refrigerated.

The fruit salad cocktail provides good amounts of antioxidants, vitamins, and minerals that help concentration and optimal brain function.

RECIPE

Morning Wake-Up Drink
Makes 1 serving

1 cup unsweetened pineapple juice (canned is okay)
1 scoop non-GMO soy or whey protein powder
½ pear, peeled
½ cup blueberries
½ to 1 scoop of Longevity Green Drink (see Appendix E, Resources) or other green powder

Optional
½ cup ice

Wash and dry all fruit. Place all ingredients in a blender or Vita-Mix, and process until smooth. This drink can be used as your first meal of the day or as a midafternoon snack. Fresh juices are best consumed within 2 to 3 hours of preparation and should be refrigerated.

Blueberries and the green powder are a brain tonic, protein powder provides high-quality energy, and pineapple juice promotes quick digestion and assimilation of all the ingredients.

CHAPTER 20

Brain: Age-Associated Memory Impairment (AAMI), Mild Cognitive Impairment (MCI), and Alzheimer's Disease

There are three basic types of memory loss: age-associated memory impairment (AAMI), mild cognitive impairment (MCI), and Alzheimer's disease (AD).

Age-associated memory impairment (AAMI) is the benign difficulty many people have with remembering names, numbers, and where they put things.

Mild cognitive impairment (MCI) is a disorder defined by its very serious loss of short-term memory. Yogesh Shah, M.D., of the Mayo Clinic, a researcher in this area, has told me of patients with MCI who forget how to get from their offices back to the parking lot. It has recently been discovered that MCI progresses to Alzheimer's disease at a rate of 12 percent per year. If we can slow this progression—and I believe we can—Alzheimer's will decrease dramatically, saving heartache and billions of health care dollars.

Alzheimer's disease results from two main pathological findings: plaques and tangles. Suffice it to say that plaques and tangles form a scar-like picture in the neuron or brain cell, which causes its death. In Alzheimer's disease there is also a reduction in memory chemicals, called neurotransmitters, the most important of which is acetylcholine. In my experience, in order to effectively prevent and treat the disease, we must target the brain cell at every level. This includes enhancing blood flow, increasing the amount of free-radical–fighting antioxidants, and replacing nutrients that make up the brain cell membrane. When doctors do this, Alzheimer's can be treated successfully in its earliest stages. Symptoms can be improved and progression slowed.

In 1929, Dr. Charles Mayo, the eminent physician, surgeon, and founder of the Mayo Clinic, said, "What can be foreseen can be prevented." If current predictions are true, and I believe they are, the number of people with Alzheimer's will soar from the current four million to over sixteen million people. Therefore, I have made it one of my missions in life to help people learn how to prevent Alzheimer's disease.

Alzheimer's is, in large measure, a disease of lifestyle, not only genetics, and nutrition plays a major part in how you live. People who eat a healthy diet are less likely to experience symptoms of dementia as they age, according to a study published in the December 2001 issue of the *European Journal of Clinical Nutrition.* By contrast, high-fat diets are linked to the development of memory loss because high fat leads to inflammation and the production of free radicals. Although it's not exactly clear how a healthy yoga nutritional therapy diet reduces the risk of Alzheimer's disease, it is thought that the vast intake of fruit and vegetables as well as the omega-3s found in fish and vegetarian substitutes are protective against brain degeneration.

DIET

The basic lower-calorie, moderate-carbohydrate and non–animal protein diet is the program of choice to lessen your risk for Alzheimer's. If a patient has Alzheimer's disease, I suggest loading up on raw or lightly steamed organic vegetables, especially spinach, and green leafy vegetables. Yellow turnips (rutabaga) are also beneficial, as are sesame seeds and sesame nut butters. Also recall that blueberries protect the brain from degeneration.

For Alzheimer's patients, salmon is the only animal protein I recommend, and only two or three times a week. Other protein sources, such as those derived from soy, can be utilized. For variety, if you enjoy the taste of Indian food, try adding curry dishes to your diet. Curry contains turmeric, which has profound antioxidant properties.

SUPPLEMENTS AND SPECIFIC NUTRIENTS

Conventional medicine approaches memory loss and dysfunction by looking for an ever-elusive magic bullet drug. I have been able to help many patients with AAMI improve their memory, those with MCI slow the progression of this condition, and those with AD reverse some of their symptoms with the following nutrients:

Primary

Everyone should take a high-potency multiple vitamin and mineral supplement as described in principle five (see page 120). In addition, for optimal brain function, I recommend taking the following nutrients:

Vitamin E: 400 to 800 I.U. per day for prevention, 800 I.U. per day for AAMI, 1,000 to 2000 I.U. per day for MCI, 2,000 I.U. per day in two divided doses for AD. Vitamin E is a potent antioxidant that helps carry oxygen to neurons in the brain and protects them from the damage of free radicals.

Coenzyme Q10: 100 mg per day for prevention and AAMI, 200 to 300 mg per day for MCI, 300 mg per day for AD. Coenzyme Q10 generates cell energy and boosts cell oxygenation.

Phosphatidylserine: 100 mg per day for protection, 200 to 300 mg per day for AAMI and MCI, 300 mg per day in three divided doses for AD. Phosphatidylserine is an interesting compound that was studied in the late 1980s and early 1990s by Thomas Crook, Ph.D., at the National Institutes of Health. Studies were also carried out at prestigious medical centers such as Stanford and Vanderbilt in America and at centers in Italy. These studies showed phosphatidylserine to be successful in reversing memory loss, but because it was derived from cow's brains, the treatment fell into disrepute after the outbreak of mad cow disease. New studies using phosphatidylserine derived from soybeans show that it improves name finding, as well as number and face recognition. One researcher stated that by his calculations, phosphatidylserine reverses brain aging by twelve years.

DHA: 100 to 1,000 mg per day. DHA is an omega-3 oil and supports optimal brain function. Anyone concerned about memory should take omega-3 supplements. I recommend at least 100 mg per day as part of a synergistic program. If you are taking omega-3 supplements alone, you may need to increase your intake to 1,000 mg a day or more.

HERBS

Primary

Ginkgo biloba: 120 mg per day for prevention and AAMI, 240 mg per day for MCI and AD. Ginkgo is an herb that is as effective as Aricept, a drug used to treat Alzheimer's. It can improve the mental functioning of patients with this disease.

Secondary

Huperzine-A: 50 to 100 mcg twice per day for MCI and AD. Huperzine-A is derived from the Chinese cub moss and is more specific in potentially treating Alzheimer's disease than any drug. It improves cognitive process and may help with short-term memory.

Vinpocetine: 2.5 to 5 mg once or twice a day for MCI and AD. Vinpocetine is derived from the periwinkle plant and is a direct brain energizer and circulation enhancer.

The dose I recommend for vinpocetine is lower than that used by other experts because my goal is protection and regeneration, not stimulation. With a higher dose, it will seem as if your brain is working better because of the jolt a high dose of this supplement gives. When the dose wears off, you may suffer a letdown, which is the mark of a stimulant. With the lower dose I recommend, there is no letdown.

Some doctors and newspaper writers have expressed concern about the possibility that the combination of vitamin E, ginkgo, and fish oil will make the blood too thin, which can lead to unwanted bleeding. While it may be remotely possible that the blood may become a bit thinner, the potential benefit is greater than that risk, which in my experience is negligible. Of course, if you are taking blood thinners such as Coumadin, you must be careful and consult your doctor.

JUICE

Brain Power Breakfast
Makes 1 serving

1 cup nonfat yogurt
½–1 tablespoon lemon juice, according to taste
⅓ cup pure water

½ scoop Longevity Green Drink (see Appendix E, Resources)
   or other green powder

Optional:
½ organic apple or ½ banana

Place all ingredients in blender. Liquefy and drink as your first
meal of the day. Fresh juices are best consumed within 2 to 3 hours
of preparation and should be refrigerated.

Yogurt provides protein and probiotic or friendly intestinal bacteria, and the green powder provides easily assimilable trace elements. Overall, this juice is an excellent brain function enhancer.

Brain Longevity Drink

½ cup organic blueberries
1 cup unsweetened pineapple juice (canned is okay)
½ scoop Longevity Green Drink (see Appendix E, Resources)
   or other green powder
1 scoop non-GMO soy or whey protein powder

Wash and dry blueberries. Place them in a blender together
with all other ingredients. Liquefy and drink as your first meal of
the day. Fresh juices are best consumed within 2 to 3 hours of
preparation and should be refrigerated.

Protein powder will give you stamina to face the day; the
Longevity Green Drink product provides trace elements and minerals; the pineapple juice is excellent as a digestion aid, diuretic,
and fat burner; and of course blueberries are a specific brain tonic.

RECIPE
Special Salmon Dinner for Your Brain
Makes 4 servings

2 medium baking potatoes
Four 5- to 6-ounce boneless, skinless salmon filet steaks
1 cup carrots, sliced
1 cup broccoli flowerets
1 cup spinach, chopped

DRESSING:
Makes ¼ cup
4 teaspoons extra virgin olive oil
½ teaspoon garlic
¼ teaspoon black pepper
2 teaspoons Braggs Liquid Aminos
1 teaspoon lemon juice
½ teaspoon thyme
1 tablespoon water

Wash and dry potatoes. Wrap potatoes in aluminum foil and bake at 375°F for 45 to 55 minutes or until soft when pierced with a fork. Broil the salmon filets for 5 minutes, then turn them over and broil for 5 more minutes, or until salmon is cooked throughout. Time may vary according to thickness of steak. Let salmon cool for 5 minutes, then cut it into long strips. Steam carrots for 5 minutes, then add broccoli and steam for another 5 minutes. Finally, add spinach and steam for another 2 minutes.

To serve, cut each potato in half, and place each half on individual dinner plates. Divide the vegetables among the plates. Arrange the salmon strips on top of vegetables. In a small bowl, whisk all dressing ingredients together, pour over dinner plate, and serve.

Salmon contains omega-3 oils, which are very important for optimal brain function. Carrots, broccoli, and spinach also support brain function with their high antioxidant content.

CHAPTER 21

Cancer Prevention and Treatment

PREVENTION

Sixty to seventy percent of all cancers are linked to lifestyle behaviors you can control—diet, physical activity, weight, and smoking. Of these lifestyle behaviors, diet is the single most important factor in cancer prevention.

Today, the ancient ideas of yoga nutritional therapy are substantiated by more than 4,500 research studies from around the globe. For cancer prevention, modern studies support a predominately plant-based diet, rich in a variety of vegetables and fruits, legumes, and grains, and the elimination of red meat from the diet. A report by Walter Willett, M.D., of Harvard Medical School, published in the *New England Journal of Medicine* in 1990 showed that eating red meat five or more times per week gave a 250 percent higher risk of developing colon cancer. This early work has been substantiated again and again. If you choose to eat animal protein, remember to limit it to no more than three times a week. Make sure it's clean protein, as discussed in the fourth principle, and no larger than a deck of cards. Better yet, use meat only as a condiment.

In cancer, absolutely the wrong signals are sent to and throughout your body. It is a disease of inflammation. Because many genes are involved in the initiation of cancer, the multiple solution approach to match this great imbalance is to consume the tens of thousands of phytonutrients that are present in a yoga nutritional therapy diet rich in vegetables and fruit. In addition, do not use tobacco of any kind. For some cancers, the effects of tobacco can overwhelm the protective effects of proper diet.

Preventing cancer of specific organs

Vegetables: Decrease the cancer risk of every organ of the body except the nasopharynx and the gallbladder.

Fruits: Decrease the cancer risk of every organ except the nasopharynx, gallbladder, liver, prostate, and kidney.

Vitamin C: In food, decreases the risk of cancer of the cervix, pancreas, stomach, lung, esophagus, bladder, and mouth.

Carotenoids: In food, decrease the cancer risk in the cervix, breast, colon, rectum, stomach, lung, bladder, and esophagus.

Selenium: In food, decreases cancer of the lung.

Whole grains: Decrease cancer of the stomach.

Nonsoluble fiber: Decreases cancers of the breast, colon, rectum, and pancreas.

Omega-3 fats: Decrease the risk of developing cancer in general, and decrease its rate of growth.

Foods, substances, and conditions that increase cancer risk

Alcohol: Breast, colon, rectum, liver, lung, esophagus, larynx, mouth.

Salt: Stomach and nasopharynx (salted fish).

Meat: Pancreas, colon, rectum, breast, prostate, kidney.

Eggs: Colon, rectum.

Animal fat: Prostate, uterus, breast, colon, rectum, lung.

Cholesterol: Pancreas, lung.

Milk and dairy products: Kidney, prostate.

Sugar: Colon, rectum.

Coffee: Bladder.

Obesity: Kidney, uterus, breast, colon, gallbladder.

Saccharine: Possibly the bladder when used in large amounts for a long time.

SUPPLEMENTS AND SPECIFIC NUTRIENTS

Primary

Everyone should take a high-potency multiple vitamin and mineral supplement as described in principle five (see page 120). In addition, for cancer prevention, I recommend taking the following nutrients:

Vitamin C: 3,000 to 10,000 mg per day according to cancer risk and tolerance to vitamin C. This vitamin is a potent anticancer agent.

Indole-3-carbinol: 150 mg three times per day. Indole-3-carbinol saturates all the tissues in the body with anticancer phytonutrients, thus preventing the development of cancer cells.

Selenium: 200 mcg per day. Selenium is a free radical hunter that protects against cancer.

Green tea extract: 100 to 300 mg per day with meals. Green tea improves cell oxygenation and also combats the effects of free radicals.

Secondary
Coenzyme Q10: 100 to 300 mg per day. Coenzyme Q10 protects cells by improving oxygenation.

SURVIVING CANCER

The only diet ever confirmed by research to reverse cancer is the macrobiotic diet, a very close cousin to yoga nutritional therapy. In fact, the recommendations for treating cancer with diet in both of these ancient healing arts is the same—a predominantly vegetarian, whole-foods diet. This type of diet has gained in popularity because of remarkable case reports of people who have attributed recovery from usually fatal cancers to dietary change.

If you have cancer, I strongly recommend the following practices:

- Make fat less than 20 percent of your diet.
- Eliminate all meat and dairy.
- Eliminate all processed foods, including artificial sweeteners.
- Make salmon and tuna about 5 percent of your diet.
- Have soy make up at least 15 percent of your diet.
- Every day, eat a serving each of broccoli, Brussels sprouts, cabbage, kale, garlic, onions, and carrots.
- Make whole grains 30 to 40 percent of your diet.

Before implementing the above, begin your healing program with a short detoxifying fast, and then eat mung beans and rice (see p. 80) as your two main meals for one week. Drink only pure water and Yogi Tea during this time.

When following this diet, you will find your tolerance to chemotherapy or radiation therapy to be greater. Your emotional well-being and overall health will also improve.

SUPPLEMENTS AND SPECIFIC NUTRIENTS

Primary

Everyone should take a high-potency multiple vitamin and mineral supplement as described in principle five (see page 120). In addition, for cancer survival, I recommend taking the following nutrients:

Vitamin C: 10,000 to 15,000 mg per day for boosting the immune system.

Secondary

MGN 3: 3 grams per day in three divided doses at mealtime for three weeks as starting dose, and then 2 grams per day in two divided doses as maintenance dose. This extract of rice bran has been demonstrated to magnify the immune response by significantly increasing the natural killer cell activity in cancer patients.

ACHH: 1,000 to 3,000 mg per day. An extract of medicinal mushrooms, ACHH helps patients survive cancer by stimulating the immune system. See Appendix E, Resources, for information about obtaining ACHH.

Inositol hexaphosphate (IP-6): 800 mg twice per day. IP-6 is an extract of brown rice that improves natural killer cell activity.

Melatonin: 3 to 20 mg under the supervision of a holistic cancer care specialist. Melatonin, the sleep hormone, is the subject of intense scientific and clinical research by several medical schools and the Cancer Treatment Centers of America. The reason is that it is a powerful antioxidant. If melatonin lives up to its promise, cancer treatment will be improved in the areas of decreased treatment toxicity, improved quality of life, and increased long-term survival. Keep checking my website at www.drdharma.com for updates on melatonin and other compounds.

Mistletoe (see also page 119): A review article on the effects of mistletoe on cancer was published in *Alternative Therapies* in 2002. The study looked at over 10,000 cancer patients and disclosed that those treated with mistletoe had better outcomes including survival. Work with your physician if you want to use mistletoe to help heal your cancer.

HERBS

Primary

Essiac tea: Drink 2 ounces three times per day at least one hour before meals for twelve consecutive weeks. Essiac tea has a long, albeit anecdotal, history in helping patients treat cancer. It is a combination of four herbs: burdock root, sorrel, slippery elm, and Indian rhubarb root. All these herbs have demonstrated anticancer activity. Essiac tea is available in health food stores.

See Appendix E, Resources, to find information on Essiac tea.

JUICE

The Immune Enhancer
Makes 1 serving

Pinch of broccoli sprouts
1 clove garlic
3 medium carrots
1 tomato
2 stalks celery

Wash and dry all the ingredients. Juice and drink. Fresh juices are best consumed within 2 to 3 hours of preparation and should be refrigerated.

This juice helps patients prevent and survive cancer by supplying a vast array of antioxidants and phytochemicals shown to have cancer-fighting properties.

Yogi Steak
Makes 6–8 wedges

1 cup yellow cornmeal
1 cup soy flour
2 tablespoons poppy seeds
½ teaspoon cayenne pepper
2 tablespoons paprika

1 tablespoon garlic powder
½ cup mustard
½ cup tamari
¼ cup water
⅔ cup broccoli florets, finely chopped
1 cup brussels sprouts, finely chopped
½ cup scallions, finely chopped
⅓ cup parsley leaves, finely chopped
2 tablespoons gingerroot, grated
3 teaspoons extra virgin olive oil
6-8 tablespoons low-fat organic yogurt
up to 1 cup of fresh sprouts per wedge

In a bowl, mix yellow cornmeal, soy flour, poppy seeds, cayenne pepper, paprika, and garlic powder. In a separate bowl, mix mustard, tamari and water, then add to the dry ingredients. Add broccoli, brussels sprouts, scallions, parsley, and gingerroot. Mix well and place in a well-oiled baking pan and pat down evenly. Spread olive oil lightly over the top and bake at 375° F for 35–45 minutes. Slice and serve hot with low-fat organic yogurt topping and sprouts.

This recipe helps patients prevent and survive cancer by supplying a vast array of antioxidants and phytochemicals shown to have cancer-fighting properties. The spices help purify the blood and clean the tissues at the cellular level. Yogi steak is an excellent bowel cleanser, gives the feeling of substantial food, and provides good protein. The yogurt aids in digestion.

If you have a condition that prevents you from eating spicy foods, or simply would like it less spicy, you can reduce the quantities of cayenne pepper, garlic powder, scallions, gingerroot, and mustard.

CHAPTER 22

Children's Health

My own two children, now grown, have never eaten meat. They both are tall, strong, and healthy. I know many other vegetarian children who are brilliant and superbly fit. They have never been sickly, have done well in school, and are very happy.

We now realize that children who grow up getting their nutrition from plant foods rather than meats have a tremendous health advantage. They are less likely to develop weight problems, diabetes, or high blood pressure. On the other hand, a childhood diet that is high in calories, animal protein, and fats may promote early menarche, which in turn leads to higher cancer rates later in life. This type of diet also promotes obesity and high blood pressure. Sixty percent of children growing up in America today are obese. Moreover, the American Heart Association notes that one in five adolescents and one in twelve children have high blood pressure. The reason may be that the average school lunch derives 37 percent of its calories from saturated fat, according to USDA surveys (www.usda.gov). By contrast, the Surgeon General states that dietary fat content over 30 percent is dangerous for children, and other health experts, myself included, call for a reduction of dietary fat for children to 20 percent or less.

DIET

A plant-based yoga nutritional therapy diet provides all the protein, vitamins, and calcium children need to grow up fit. Vegetables and legumes provide a healthy source of calcium along with many other nutritional advantages. This proven medical fact led the prominent pediatrician Dr. Benjamin Spock to say that even cow's milk consumption by children was unnecessary.

If you are concerned about calcium, please realize that 8 ounces of calcium-fortified orange juice has more calcium (300 mg) than 8 ounces of milk. Some soy and rice milks have calcium as well as vitamins A, D, and B_{12} added, providing the same amount of nutrients as cow's milk without the high fat content, antibiotics, and hormones. Here is a list of plant foods high in calcium:

Almonds, ½ cup	166 mg
Bok choy, 1 cup	250 mg
Broccoli, 1 cup	178 mg
Collard greens, 1 cup	226 mg
Figs, 5 medium	258 mg
Kelp, 1 tablespoon	156 mg
Pinto beans, 1 cup	82 mg
Sesame tahini, 1 tablespoon	64 mg
Sweet potato, 1 cup	70 mg
Tofu, ½ cup	188 mg
Wax beans, 1 cup	174 mg

If you still choose to have milk in your child's diet, remember to at least make it organic.

Mother Teresa once said, "The way you can help heal the world is to start with your own family." A yoga nutritional therapy dietary program is healthy for your children and your family. Beyond that, it will help you take one small step toward creating a better world for the next generations.

SUPPLEMENTS AND SPECIFIC NUTRIENTS

Primary

The only nutrient that may be difficult for children to obtain on a pure vegetarian or vegan diet is vitamin B_{12}. Although cereals are fortified with vitamin B_{12} and other vitamins, I suggest that vegetarian children and teenagers take a multivitamin and mineral supplement that contains vitamin B_{12}. Meat-eating children usually have no difficulty obtaining enough vitamin B_{12}. I recommend that all children, however, take a multiple vitamin and mineral supplement as insurance against today's poor diet and the stresses of growing up. You can find children's vitamins in your local health food store.

HERBS

In general, I do not use herbal therapy for healthy children.

RECIPES
Celery Raisin Drink
Makes 1 serving

> 2 stalks celery
> 1 handful raisins

Wash and dry the celery. Place the raisins in a pan, and cover with 1 or 2 inches of purified water. Bring to a boil, and cook for a few minutes more until the water is colored by the raisins. While the raisins are boiling, put the celery through a juicer. Remove raisins from heat, and strain the raisin water into a cup. Mix raisin water and celery juice together, cool, and serve. For very young children, dilute by half with water. The celery raisin drink is best consumed within 2 to 3 hours of preparation and should be refrigerated. You can use the raisins as a snack later or eat them in cereal. Celery raisin drink helps to calm and relax children by balancing the body's chemistry. Celery is a natural relaxant, and raisins provide vitamins and minerals.

Date Milk
Makes 1 serving

> ½ cup pure water
> 1 cup organic milk
> 6 pitted dates, sliced in half

Simmer ingredients together on low heat for 20 minutes, or until the milk is a pinkish color and the dates are breaking down. Stir occasionally. Strain before serving. The soothing, delicious taste of date milk helps wean babies from breastfeeding while providing nourishment to replace mother's milk. But date milk isn't just for babies—it is a very nutritious, youth-maintaining beverage for people of all ages. It gives energy to the body and helps to ward off colds. Date milk is very good to drink when you are recovering from a fever or the flu.

CHAPTER 23

Chronic Fatigue

Chronic fatigue is a terrible problem in our society today. Although there is scientific evidence that tracks the cause of chronic fatigue to the Epstein-Barr virus, I have had many healing partners who were free of viral infection but still had severe chronic fatigue syndrome.

For example, there was my patient Marilyn, a forty-six-year-old executive in the apparel business. Constant travel and the financial pressures of her business were wearing her out. These stressors were also placing quite a bit of strain on her relationship with her husband and two teenaged children. Fortunately, they were a committed family.

I diagnosed Marilyn with chronic fatigue syndrome. Like many of her peers, Marilyn had been struggling hard for success and was now paying an enormous price in terms of her health. It was clear that too much time on the road and the accompanying difficulty in finding good, nutritious food while traveling had damaged her health.

To combat Marilyn's chronic fatigue, I prescribed a complete yoga nutritional therapy program. What restored her zest and vitality the most, however, was a special antifatigue drink called the yoga nutritional therapy energy plus drink (see page 202). It is easy to make, tastes great, and works fast.

After only a few days of using the drink, Marilyn felt fantastic. Color returned to her cheeks, and her energy was great. Now if she feels fatigued she enjoys the drink for a few days, and her energy comes roaring back. "The best thing about this simple little concoction, Dr. Dharma," she told me, "is that it's amazingly potent. I mean, it really works!"

DIET

In addition, I had Marilyn follow a mung bean and rice diet (see page 80) for a week. Thereafter, she embarked on a yoga nutritional therapy diet, rich in energy-giving vegetables, fruit, some grains and beans, and lower-fat sources of protein such as soy. She also ate salmon twice weekly.

SUPPLEMENTS AND SPECIFIC NUTRIENTS

Primary

Every person with chronic fatigue should take a high-potency multiple vitamin and mineral supplement as described in the fifth principle (see page 120), and the following specific nutrients:

Vitamin C: 3,000 to 9,000 mg per day as tolerated. Vitamin C has an antiviral effect and boosts energy.

Coenzyme Q10: 100 mg per day. Coenzyme Q10 enhances the functioning of the immune system.

Alpha-lipoic acid: 100 mg per day. Alpha-lipoic acid helps cells to metabolize energy and acts as a powerful antioxidant.

DHEA: 25 to 100 mg per day. DHEA has been shown to increase energy levels and mood in people with chronic fatigue syndrome. As with any other hormone, you should take DHEA only under a doctor's supervision.

Secondary

N-*acetylcysteine (NAC)*: 250 mg per day. NAC is a powerful detoxifier and acts against agents that suppress the immune system.

Germanium: Although the dose response varies considerably, the average reported dose is 500 mg sublingually (under the tongue) twice per day. Germanium is an antiviral nutrient that stimulates the body's production of interferon, a natural immune system enhancer. It works in concert with coenzyme Q10.

HERBS

Primary

Ginseng: 150 mg twice per day. Ginseng fights against weakness and provides extra energy.

Secondary

Ginkgo biloba: 120 mg in the morning. Ginkgo boosts circulation and brain function.

Also drink as much Yogi Tea as you like. It contains cardamom, ginger, and cloves. Ginseng, ginkgo biloba, and Yogi Tea each reverse fatigue and provide energy.

JUICE

Energy Plus
Makes 1 serving

½ apple
¼ cup blueberries
1 banana
1 cup unsweetened pineapple juice
1 scoop non-GMO soy or whey protein powder
¼ scoop Longevity Green Drink (see Appendix E, Resources)
    or other green powder

Wash and dry apple and blueberries. Peel the banana and place it in blender with all the remaining ingredients. Blend well before drinking. Fresh juices are best consumed within 2 to 3 hours of preparation and should be refrigerated.

Bananas are rich in potassium, important for energy and muscle function. Blueberries are rich in antioxidants and are a brain tonic. Pineapple juice promotes optimal digestion. Protein powder provides sustained levels of energy, and the green powder is an important source of trace elements.

RECIPE

Yoga nutritional therapy Energy-Plus Drink
Makes 1 serving

½ cup pure water
½ or 1 teaspoon turmeric powder
8 to 12 ounces milk or milk substitute
3 to 5 dates

1 tablespoon edible almond oil
1 teaspoon honey (optional)

Place water and turmeric in a pot. Boil until the turmeric has a pastelike consistency, thick and viscous, then add 8 to 12 ounces of milk. Stir well and bring to a boil. In the meantime, chop 3 to 5 dates, and add to the milk. Let boil for 3 minutes, then let cool down for a few minutes.

In a blender, place almond oil, the milk/date mixture, and honey, and blend. This drink is best consumed within 2 to 3 hours of preparation and should be refrigerated.

Variation for women: Blend 8 blanched almonds together with the other ingredients. Almonds help sustain calcium levels, which affect the regulation of the menstrual cycle.

Variation for men: Add a pinch of saffron to the turmeric at the very beginning, then follow the recipe. Saffron helps sustain potency.

Drink once a day first thing in the morning or in the evening at bedtime. This recipe boosts the immune system and is an excellent source of protein and iron.

CHAPTER 24

Chronic Pain: Arthritis, Backache or Sciatica, Fibromyalgia, and Headache

The great physician and humanitarian Dr. Albert Schweitzer once said that living with chronic pain could be worse than death itself. Many people with chronic pain can probably agree with him. Being in pain day after day brings you down and saps your strength, spirit, hope, personality, and ability to love.

The good news is that life need not be a painful struggle. I have helped hundreds of people heal from chronic pain over the length of my twenty-five-year medical career. The nutritional information I present in this chapter on pain can help you feel better.

DIET

My friend Andrew started out as a patient. His acupuncturist asked me to consult with him because of polymyositis, an excruciatingly painful inflammatory and debilitating illness. This disease was eating up his muscles. His conventional doctor had him taking several drugs, including the immune suppressant prednisone, in an effort to reduce his inflammation. It wasn't helping. In fact, his doctor told him that he had six months to live with or without the drug.

The first thing I did was prescribe a low-inflammation diet consisting of fresh vegetable juices, steamed vegetables, fruits, grains, soy, and a hearty nine-grain bread. I also had him begin every day with a period of medical meditation. That was over six years ago. Today he does not take any medication except a sleep aid, and he has energy enough to maintain his thriving businesses.

I can tell you without qualification that what you eat will help you reduce your pain. The main principle is to eat foods that relieve inflammation. They are the foods I suggested to Andrew: vegetables, fruits, grains, and soy. Fish such as salmon, which is high in anti-inflammatory omega-3s, is also quite beneficial. Andrew didn't care much for fish but felt he needed more protein, so we selected clean turkey. It has worked well.

Another way to eliminate pain is to eat foods that boost the level of the pain-fighting hormone serotonin in your brain. Serotonin is manufactured by the body from a partial protein or amino acid called tryptophan. This amino acid is found in many foods, including soy, turkey, chicken, halibut, beans, and cheddar cheese. Be careful to limit the amount of cheddar cheese, however, because it's high in fat. To get the most benefit from your dietary change and to build up your levels of serotonin, eat the starch in your meal, such as whole grain pasta, first. Then eat the protein.

Next, avoid harmful pro-inflammatory cooking oils such as corn oil, safflower oil, cooked sesame oil, and canola oil. Instead, use only extra virgin olive oil or ghee.

Finally, avoid hypoglycemia (low blood sugar). You can do so by eating enough at mealtime and having healthful snacks throughout the day. Of course, you want to avoid processed food snacks because they are high in simple sugar, which will actually defeat the purpose of avoiding low blood sugar. Why? Because snacks high in sugar, although they may give you an initial sugar high, will subsequently lower your blood sugar and make you feel very tired. This will make your pain worse.

SUPPLEMENTS AND SPECIFIC NUTRIENTS

Primary

Everyone with a chronic pain condition should take a high-potency multiple vitamin and mineral supplement, as described in the fifth principle (see page 120). In addition, the following nutrients should be added to your daily diet:

Phosphatidylserine: 100 to 300 mg per day. Phosphatidylserine enhances brain function, which helps control chronic pain.

Magnesium: At least 200 to 300 mg per day. Magnesium is usually part of your multivitamin, but if your muscles are tight, you may need more.

Magnesium is considered necessary for appropriate functioning of all muscles and alleviates muscle pain.

DHEA: 50 to 100 mg per day to brighten mood and increase brain function. As with any other hormone, you should take DHEA only under a doctor's supervision.

Secondary
Tryptophan: Start with 250 to 500 mg per day and work up to 3,000 mg per day. Take the higher doses only under the care of a physician. Tryptophan raises serotonin levels.

HERBS

Primary
Ginseng: 750 to 1,500 mg of Siberian ginseng per day increases energy.

Turmeric: 100 to 200 mg per day. Turmeric has anti-inflammatory properties. It may also be taken as spice in food.

Ginger: 1,000 mg per day in divided doses. Ginger may also be added as spice in food. Ginger reduces inflammation and stimulates blood flow.

Secondary
Ginkgo biloba: 120 mg per day increases circulation and enhances brain function.

Boswellian: 300 mg per day. Boswellian is an ancient yoga nutritional therapy from the *Boswellia serrata* tree. It helps reduce inflammation and reinstate the blood vessels around irritated connective tissue.

ARTHRITIS

Nearly 60 million Americans have arthritis. Yet, by following a few simple dietary guidelines, many could avoid such suffering.

Foods in the nightshade family, such as tomatoes, peppers, eggplant, and some citrus fruit, aggravate arthritis and should be avoided. Also, eliminate from your diet refined flour and white sugar. Instead, follow all the yoga nutritional therapy principles, and make the transition to a plant-based diet. All the dietary advice given under general chronic pain also holds for arthritis.

I have seen remarkable pain relief in patients with osteoarthritis, the wear-and-tear type, and in those with rheumatoid arthritis who follow the short detoxifying program outlined in the first principle (see page 70).

SUPPLEMENTS AND SPECIFIC NUTRIENTS

Primary

All people with arthritis should take a high-potency multiple vitamin and mineral supplement, as explained in the fifth principle (see page 120). Also, in addition to the nutrients suggested for chronic pain, other very useful nutrients for arthritis are these:

SAM-e (S-adenosylmethionine): 600 to 1,200 mg per day. SAM-e is very effective for generating new cartilage and reducing pain. It also has been shown to improve mood. If gastrointestinal upset occurs, reduce the dose until the upset subsides.

Glucosamine sulfate (GS): 500 mg three times per day. GS is superior to conventional medicines such as ibuprofen and the selective cox-2 inhibitors such as Vioxx. In a study published in *The Lancet* in 2001, 212 patients were divided into two groups; one received GS, the other a placebo. The patients receiving GS had a remarkable outcome. They had less pain and also showed no loss of joint space, which is a hallmark of progressive arthritis. What's more, the GS worked without the potential for side effects such as stomachache or severe life-threatening gastrointestinal bleeding, which can occur without warning in patients taking drugs such as Vioxx.

Chondroitin sulfate: 800 to 1,200 mg per day. Chondroitin sulfate has powerful anti-inflammatory activity and can prevent or delay the progression of osteoarthritis.

Additional special supplements for rheumatoid arthritis include the following:

Primary

Ginger: 500 to 1,000 mg per day. Ginger has anti-inflammatory properties.

Secondary

Borage oil: 1,400 mg per day. Borage oil supplies an excellent amount of anti-inflammatory nutrients.

Black currant seed oil: 10 grams per day. Black currant seed has anti-inflammatory properties.

BACKACHE OR SCIATICA

Following the yoga nutritional therapy program and all the seven principles will go a long way toward ending your back pain. The reason is that you will reduce painful inflammation and lose weight, removing some burden from the back muscles and the spine.

SUPPLEMENTS AND SPECIFIC NUTRIENTS

Everyone with back pain should take a high-potency multiple vitamin and mineral supplement, as explained in the fifth principle (see page 120), plus the following nutrients, in addition to those already outlined for chronic pain:

Calcium: 1,000 to 2,500 mg per day. Calcium is important for strong bones.

Vitamin C: 1000 to 2000 mg per day beyond that found in your multiple vitamin. Vitamin C decreases inflammation by reducing free radicals.

Vitamin D: 500 to 800 mg per day when you can't get at least half an hour of direct sunshine. Vitamin D facilitates the absorption of calcium.

FIBROMYALGIA

The pieces of the puzzle known as fibromyalgia are finally starting to come together. A main key to the mystery now appears to be low levels of the hormone serotonin. The best way to nutritionally boost your level of serotonin is to increase your body's supply of tryptophan, the building block from which serotonin is made. The best way to increase your level of tryptophan, in addition to eating soy, turkey, chicken, halibut, beans, and cheddar cheese, is to take 5-hydroxytryptophan supplements (5-HTP) daily. Following an anti-inflammatory yoga nutritional therapy diet is, of course, also crucially important in reducing the symptoms of fibromyalgia.

SUPPLEMENTS AND SPECIFIC NUTRIENTS

Primary

Everyone should take a high-potency multiple vitamin and mineral supplement, as explained in the fifth principle (see page 120). In addition to the nutrients already suggested for chronic pain, I recommend the following nutrients for those with fibromyalgia:

5-HTP: 100 mg three times per day. You can find 5-HTP in any health food store. There are no contraindications and no side effects. Pycnogenol, a nutrient available in most stores, helps your body metabolize 5-HTP to tryptophan and may be taken along with your 5-HTP supplement.

Magnesium: 300 to 500 mg per day is very important to help keep your muscles relaxed.

Coenzyme Q10: 100 to 300 mg per day in three divided doses. Coenzyme Q10 improves cell oxygenation.

DHEA: 50 to 100 mg per day has been shown to decrease pain and increase energy in patients with fibromyalgia. As with any other hormone, you should take DHEA only under a doctor's supervision.

Secondary

Longevity Green Drink (see Appendix E, Resources) or other green powder: ½ to 1 full scoop per day. Green drinks have an assortment of micronutrients that increase energy levels in people with fibromyalgia.

HEADACHE

All types of headache pain can be helped by following a yoga nutritional therapy diet. A short detoxifying program, including a juice fast, will usually help identify food allergies, which may be responsible for your headache. Beyond that, it appears that low levels of the hormone serotonin are, in large measure, responsible for the genesis of headache pain.

The worst offenders in causing headache are caffeine and some citrus fruits. The artificial sweetener aspartame contains the amino acid phenylalanine, which constricts blood vessels, thus bringing on headaches. You should eliminate it completely from your diet. You must also stop eating processed foods or cured meats such as hot dogs or bacon, because they contain sodium nitrates, which also can bring on headaches.

Meat, milk products, and eggs trigger migraines in many people. An additive that often triggers migraines is monosodium glutamate (MSG), which is found in Chinese food and many packaged, processed foods. MSG is also genetically modified. It may also be referred to as "hydrogenated vegetable protein," "natural preservatives," or "seasonings."

SUPPLEMENTS AND SPECIFIC NUTRIENTS

Primary

Everyone should take a high-potency multiple vitamin and mineral supplement, as explained in the fifth principle (see page 120). In addition to nutrients recommended for chronic pain, I suggest the following supplements for persons with headache:

5-HTP: 100 mg three times per day. 5-HTP has shown positive results with migraines. 5-HTP increases the levels of serotonin, the pain-fighting and feel-good hormone.

Secondary

Magnesium: 200 mg per day. Although this amount may be found in your daily multiple vitamin and mineral supplement, it is often helpful to take an additional 200 mg during the day, especially if you are under stress. Magnesium relaxes the muscles and eases muscular tension.

Niacin: 500 mg at the start of a headache increases blood flow to all capillaries and may help relieve headaches.

HERBS

Primary

Ginger: One 500-mg tablet, or drink a cup of ginger tea per day. Ginger fights inflammation and stimulates circulation.

Feverfew: 150 to 1,000 mg per day in two divided doses. Feverfew can be found in most health food stores. Feverfew may act as a blood thinner, so if you are taking coumadin, discuss taking feverfew with your health care practitioner.

Feverfew is very effective in the prevention and reversal of headaches, especially migraines. Studies since the 1980s have demonstrated that this herb has excellent anti-inflammatory and serotonin-balancing effects. It may also affect the metabolism of melatonin. Feverfew needs to be taken every day for at least a month to be optimally effective.

Secondary
Milk thistle: 500 mg twice per day. There are no side effects or contraindications to milk thistle, which detoxifies the liver. In yoga nutritional therapy, liver toxins are said to cause headaches.

JUICE

Pain Relief Shake
Makes 1 serving

1 small red apple
1 plum
¼ cup blueberries or cherries
1 teaspoon flaxseed oil
juice of 1 lemon
¼ scoop Longevity Green Drink (see Appendix E, Resources)
    or other green powder
1 cup of ice or pure water

Wash and dry the apple, plum, and berries. Place them in a blender with remaining ingredients. Blend well and drink. Fresh juices are best consumed within 2 to 3 hours of preparation and should be refrigerated.

The pain relief shake supports immune function by providing numerous antioxidants, omega-3 oils, and trace elements.

RECIPE

Mung beans and rice (see page 80) is excellent as an anti-inflammatory chronic pain staple. You can also try the following unique recipe.

The Pain Cure Vegetarian Sushi
Makes 15 pieces

½ cup millet
⅔ cup quinoa
2 cups pure water

1 tablespoon lemon juice, fresh
1 tablespoon brown rice syrup
1 organic carrot
½ cucumber
1 celery stalk
1 green onion
½ avocado
1-inch piece of fresh ginger, peeled and grated
4 sheets of nori (toasted)

DIPPING SAUCE: *Mix together in a small bowl*

1 tablespoon Braggs Liquid Aminos
½ to 1 tablespoon fresh grated gingerroot
1 tablespoon water
½ teaspoon honey or brown rice syrup
1½ sprigs scallions, finely minced

Rinse millet and quinoa, then pour into boiling water. Under medium high heat, bring back to a boil, then simmer for 15 minutes or until the water is absorbed. Allow to cool. Mix lemon juice and brown rice syrup into the grains. Cut the carrot, cucumber, celery, onion, and avocado into julienne strips lengthwise. Steam the carrot and ginger pieces for 5 minutes, and allow to cool.

Prepare a bowl of cold, salted water to wet your fingers so that the grain and nori won't stick to them. Working on a cutting board, take a damp cloth and gently moisten both sides of the nori sheet. Place several tablespoons of grain on the nori sheet. Smooth the grain evenly over the sheet to a thickness of ¼ to ⅜ inch, so that it covers all except the last inch or two farthest away from you. Arrange the vegetables in two or three horizontal rows on top of the grain. You may mix them together, but keep them in straight rows to make rolling easier. Tuck over the edge closest to you and keep rolling. When you come to the end of the grain, lightly moisten the last inch or so of bare nori, and let the pressure of the roll and your hands seal it. With a sharp knife cut the roll into five or six pieces. Repeat for the remaining nori sheets. Serve arranged on a tray with dipping sauce. Makes 15 pieces.

Note: If nori is not toasted, hold it over a gas flame or roast in a saucepan until it turns green. When it is not toasted, it is much tougher and may crumble when you try to eat it.

This recipe, although it appears daunting, is actually quite easy. It just takes a little time and effort, but it will be very healing for your chronic pain. Millet and quinoa have a good protein content, are very easily digestible, and have a very calming effect on inflammation. All the vegetables in this recipe are rich in powerful antioxidants; help detoxify the body, thus further reducing inflammation; and provide good omega-3 fats and vitamins.

CHAPTER 25

Cleansing and Detoxification

Cleansing your body is essential if you wish to be healthy. I recommend that you undergo a cleansing and detoxification diet once or twice a year. Cleansing rids your body of toxins from air and water pollution, stress, and poor nutrition. It also helps rejuvenate your cells.

DIET

Foods that are known to be cleansing are oranges or orange juice with its own pulp, for its high content of beta-carotene and fiber; garlic, for its antibacterial properties; beets, for their liver detoxification action; apples, for their high fiber content and soothing effects on the gastrointestinal system; grapes, for their high antioxidant, mineral, and fiber content; parsley, for its kidney detoxification properties; watermelon, for its high fiber content and kidney detoxification properties; and wheat grass, for its liver detoxification property.

There are many ways to begin a cleansing and detoxifying program. One easy way is to do a short juice fast followed by a monodiet. Take it at your own pace, be open and patient, and you will see fantastic results. For more information on fasting and detoxification, please see chapter 8, page 70.

SUPPLEMENTS AND SPECIFIC NUTRIENTS

I usually recommend stopping all vitamins except vitamin C during a cleansing program. Because of its strong immune enhancing properties, vitamin C can be taken at a dose of 3,000 to 6,000 mg per day. Please continue to take your prescription medicines.

HERBS

Secondary
Milk thistle: 320 mg a day with juices or meals. Milk thistle helps detoxify the liver and may have a mild laxative effect.

JUICE

If you just want to start your cleansing program without going on a fast, try incorporating these three juices into your daily diet:

Detox juice #1
⅓ cup fresh grapefruit juice, ⅓ cup fresh apple juice, ⅓ cup fresh carrot juice, combined, four times a day.

Grapefruit helps detoxify the liver, apple helps the digestion, and carrot provides beta-carotene, important for the eyes, pancreas, and spleen.

Detox juice #2
1 cup of fresh orange juice. Orange juice provides optimal levels of vitamins, especially beta-carotene.

Detox juice #3
1 cup of fresh celery juice. Celery juice is a natural relaxant and helps cleanse the stomach and colon.

Fresh juices are best consumed within 2 to 3 hours of preparation and should be refrigerated.

RECIPE

The melon fast
To begin the fast: Eat only cantaloupes for three days. The following three days, eat only watermelons, followed by three days of papayas, followed by three days of lukewarm lemon-honey water. On the last day, drink only water at room temperature. Then reverse the diet, starting with one day of lukewarm water, followed by three days of lemon-honey water, three days of papayas, three days of watermelons, and finally three days of cantaloupes.

To break the fast: First eat fruits for one or two days, then add yogurt and vegetables for two or three days, and finally start a complete diet.

Note: If you want to try a shorter fast, you can follow the same protocol outlined above but reduce each three-day period to one day.

The melon fast is excellent for a total cleanse. Cantaloupes are warming and have a mild laxative effect. Watermelon cleanses the liver and kidneys. Papayas help the intestines and digestion. The lemon-honey water rids the body of excess mucus.

I recommend this program during the summer, when the temperature is warm and these fruits are in season. This fast is great for losing weight. It will cleanse the large and small intestines, replace all the bodily fluids, and provide a detoxifying break for all your organs. During this fasting time, massage almond oil into your skin every day, drink plenty of water, and do yoga and meditation regularly to help your body go through the cleanse. Also, take vitamin C and milk thistle during this time to enhance the results of the fast.

As with any other fast, if you have any medical condition you should consult your doctor before fasting. If you feel excessively weak, then break the fast as described above.

CHAPTER 26

Depression

Between 1987 and 1997, the number of Americans treated for depression soared from 1.7 million to 6.3 million. In the same time period, the proportion of those receiving antidepressants doubled, according to the January 2002 edition of the *Journal of the American Medical Association*. In the aftermath of September 11, 2001, the number of depressed people rose even more, with a reported surge in sleeplessness, anxiety, decreased energy, substance abuse, eating disorders, and other unhealthy behaviors.

Antidepressant medication combined with talk therapy clearly helps, but it does not provide the true long-term solution. For that to occur, the problems underlying depression must be addressed, and holistic solutions, such as nutritional biochemistry, must be implemented.

Depression results from an upset in the fragile balance of the brain chemicals that control mood. It is a whole-body disease that can twist the way you think and behave, often damaging your physical health as well as your emotions. It's a powerful condition that can leave you unable to work, maintain relationships, or deal with other responsibilities.

The human brain has an average of fifteen billion cells called neurons. Many other cells fill the spaces between these neurons, and miles and miles of blood vessels nourish all the brain cells. Brain tissue is only about 3 percent of your body weight, yet it requires 25 percent of circulating blood. Beyond that, the brain requires specific nutrients that, when provided, can reverse fatigue, irritability, anxiety, and depression.

DIET

Glucose is the brain's main fuel. If glucose levels decrease, you may feel tired, depressed, or incapable of thinking clearly. A yoga nutritional therapy diet with plenty of raw fruits and vegetables, plus soybeans and soy products, helps keep your neurochemicals balanced. Whole grains, nuts, seeds, and legumes should also be added. Complex carbohydrates induce a feeling of relaxation, whereas high-protein meals stimulate alertness. Stay away from diet sodas and other products containing aspartame, which can block the formation of serotonin, the feel-good chemical. Keep away from foods high in saturated fats, such as red meat and fried foods, which can cause mental fatigue. These foods interfere with blood flow to the brain. Also avoid sugar, alcohol, caffeine, and processed foods.

SUPPLEMENTS AND SPECIFIC NUTRIENTS

Primary

Everyone should take a high-potency multiple vitamin and mineral supplement, as explained in the fifth principle (see page 120). I also recommend the following vitamins and nutrients for depression:

Vitamin B_{12}: 500 mcg of sublingual (under the tongue) vitamin B_{12} twice per day. Vitamin B_{12} acts as a mild mental stimulator.

Vitamin C: Start with 1,000 mg twice per day, and gradually increase the dosage to 3,000 mg twice per day. Vitamin C increases physical and mental energy.

DHEA: 25 to 100 mg per day has been shown to enhance mood and mental energy. As with any other hormone, you should take DHEA only under a doctor's supervision.

Omega-3 fatty acids: 1,000 mg per day to optimize nervous system function.

Secondary

Vitamin B_3: Start with 25 mg per day, and gradually increase the dose to 300 to 400 mg per day. Vitamin B_3 increases mental energy.

Vitamin B_5: Take up to 250 mg per day to increase mental energy.

Pregnenolone: 10 to 100 mg per day. Pregnenolone is associated with improved brain function and helps mood and thinking.

HERBS

Primary

Hypericum (St. John's wort): 300 mg three times per day. St. John's wort raises levels of serotonin naturally. Overall, 60 to 80 percent of people respond to St. John's wort with some improvement in mood.

Secondary

Ginseng: 150 to 300 mg per day. Ginseng enhances overall physical and mental health.

Ginkgo biloba: 80 mg three times per day. Ginkgo increases blood flow to the brain and has a mild stimulating effect.

JUICE

Depression Buster
Makes 1 serving

1 banana
4 or 5 dates
1 cup orange juice (canned is okay)
¼ to ½ scoop Longevity Green Drink (see Appendix E, Resources) or other green powder

Peel the banana and blend with remaining ingredients. Drink immediately. Fresh juices are best consumed within 2 to 3 hours of preparation and should be refrigerated.

Bananas, dates, and orange juice are rich in vitamins and minerals that help prevent and decrease depression. The green powder is rich in minerals and trace elements that benefit the brain.

RECIPE

Martín's Salmon Plate
Makes 2 servings

2 ½-lb fresh salmon fillets
½ gallon pure water
2 carrots, peeled and julienned
2 tablespoons parsley, finely chopped

½ onion, sliced as rings
1 red pepper, thinly sliced
2 medium cloves garlic, minced
4 slices lemon
½ tablespoon lemon juice
⅛ teaspoon sea salt
⅛ teaspoon black pepper

Optional:
2 teaspoons flaxseed oil

Rinse salmon in cold water. In the meantime, bring water to a boil. In a large strainer, arrange food in three layers. The first layer is made of half the carrot, parsley, onion, red pepper, garlic, and the lemon slices. The second layer is made of salmon fillets, sprinkled with lemon juice, salt, and pepper. The third layer is the remaining half of the vegetables.

Place strainer above the boiling water. Cover and let steam salmon until cooked, approximately 10 minutes, or until salmon is cooked throughout.

To add more flavor, you can add additional lemon juice, red pepper, garlic, and black pepper to boiling water.

Arrange the top layer of vegetables on one plate, and place one fillet in the center; prepare the second plate in the same way, sprinkle with flaxseed oil and serve.

Salmon is an important source of healthy nutrients for the body and the brain. It provides optimal energy and nutrients that restore proper chemical balance.

CHAPTER 27

Diabetes

The goal of treating diabetes is to stabilize blood sugar levels, and to prevent vascular damage and some of the other serious complications that can result from diabetes. A combination of herbs and a healthy diet, along with lifestyle changes, can be quite helpful.

DIET

The yoga nutritional therapy diet, containing moderate to high protein, low fat, and reasonable amounts of complex carbohydrates, is excellent for diabetes. Soy protein, mung beans, and rice provide a strong foundation. Fish is also an important part of this diet because the omega-3 fats help the body use insulin. The yoga nutritional therapy diet also limits the heart problems associated with diabetes.

SUPPLEMENTS AND SPECIFIC NUTRIENTS

Primary

Everyone should take a high-potency multiple vitamin and mineral supplement, as explained in the fifth principle (see page 120). In addition, for diabetes, I recommend the following:

Fish oil: 1,200 mg twice per day. Fish oil is a good source of protein.

Vitamin C: 2,000 to 3,000 mg per day. Vitamin C may slow or prevent problems that arise from diabetes.

Brewer's yeast: 3 tablespoons per day. Brewer's yeast is a good source of vitamin B, which regulates glucose utilization.

Chromium: 200 mcg twice per day. Chromium improves glucose tolerance.

Coenzyme Q10: 100 to 200 mg per day. Coenzyme Q10 stabilizes blood sugar levels.

Secondary
Evening primrose oil: 2,000 mg twice per day. Primrose oil helps prevent hardening of the arteries and high blood pressure.

Grapeseed extract: 100 mg twice per day. Grapeseed extract helps maintain proper oxygen delivery in all organs, helps tonify the pancreas, and helps regulate insulin secretion.

Niacin: 800 mg twice per day. Niacin helps with the metabolism of carbohydrates, fat, and proteins.

HERBS
Primary
Bilberry: 250 mg per day for vision protection.

Secondary
Ginger: 500 to 2,000 mg per day. Ginger stimulates blood flow.

JUICE

Veggie Diabetes Drink
Makes 1 serving

2 stalks celery
3 beet greens
½ green pepper
1 tomato

Wash and dry all the ingredients, then juice them. Fresh juices are best consumed within 2 or 3 hours of preparation and should be refrigerated.

These vegetables provide good amounts of vitamins and minerals that are beneficial for patients with diabetes.

RECIPE

Malcolm's Veggie Chili and Tofu
Makes 4 servings

2 cloves garlic, minced
8 ounces firm tofu, crumbled
1 14 ½-ounce can chopped tomatoes
1 15-ounce can red kidney beans, drained
2 large carrots, thinly sliced
1 medium sized green pepper, chopped
½ to 1 teaspoon chili powder
1 teaspoon ground cumin
salt and pepper to taste

SALAD:
6 cups butter lettuce

BALSAMIC VINEGAR DRESSING:
¼ teaspoon minced garlic
¼ cup balsamic vinegar
¼ teaspoon dried oregano
¼ teaspoon dried basil
⅛ teaspoon sea salt
⅛ teaspoon ground black pepper
½ teaspoon honey
1 teaspoon Dijon mustard
1 tablespoon extra virgin olive oil

Heat the oil, and sauté the onion and garlic for 3 or 4 minutes. Stir in the tofu and cook for 5 minutes to lightly brown the tofu. Add tomatoes, kidney beans, carrots, and green pepper. Saute for 5 minutes over medium heat. Add the chili, cumin, salt, and pepper. Simmer slowly over low heat for 30 minutes. Add a little water if it becomes too dry.

Wash and dry the butter lettuce, then chop in bite-size pieces. In a small bowl, whisk together the garlic, vinegar, oregano, basil, salt, pepper, honey, and mustard. Slowly pour in the olive oil and whisk to slightly thicken. Toss the salad and let sit for 10 minutes before serving.

This recipe provides optimal nutrition and a good balance of protein and carbohydrates while respecting the carbohydrate restrictions that diabetic persons must follow. For the exchange system used by diabetes patients, each ½ cup of the chili equals one carbohydrate choice and one protein choice.

CHAPTER 28

Digestive Health: Gallbladder, Stomach (Acid and Ulcers), Liver, and Colon (Inflammation, Constipation, and Hemorrhoids)

The yoga nutritional therapy diet is ideal for maintaining maximum digestive health. The mung beans and rice recipe (see page 80) provides a good natural approach because its many nutrients are easy to digest and assimilate into the body.

As you may know, the gastrointestinal system is composed of the following organs: stomach, liver, gallbladder, pancreas, small intestine, and large intestine. In fact, good digestion actually begins in your mouth because of the enzymes that are secreted when you look at, smell, and even think about your food.

GALLBLADDER

The gallbladder is a little green organ that sits underneath your liver. It secretes bile acids into your small intestine; the acids then mix with pancreatic juices and help begin the assimilation process of food.

Diet

Poor digestion and heavy, greasy foods contribute to gallbladder disease. Eat a wide variety of fresh vegetables, and reduce your total fat intake to improve this condition.

Yoga nutritional therapy foods that are especially beneficial for gall-bladder disease are pears, which help dissolve gallstones, and horseradish, which is a gallbladder and liver cleanser.

SUPPLEMENTS AND SPECIFIC NUTRIENTS

Primary

Everyone should take a high-potency multiple vitamin and mineral supplement, as explained in the fifth principle (see p. 120). In addition, to support the gallbladder, I recommend the following nutrients:

Essential fatty acid complex: 1,000 mg per day. Essential fatty acids help repair and prevent gallstones.

Digestive enzymes: 1 to 2 capsules or tablets with each meal, depending on what supplement you use. These enzymes help with digestion if too little bile is secreted from the gallbladder.

Secondary

Vitamin C: 1,000 to 3,000 mg per day. Some studies link vitamin C deficiency to gallstones.

HERBS

Primary

Turmeric: 100 mg three times per day. Turmeric is a natural anti-inflammatory.

Secondary

Alfalfa: 1,000 to 2,000 mg per day. Alfalfa helps cleanse the liver and gallbladder.

STOMACH (ACID AND ULCERS)

In addition to nutritional or metabolic causes, gastric and duodenal ulcers can be the result of chronic mental and nervous stress. Ulcers can also be caused by infection with *Helicobacter pylori* bacteria combined with stomach acid.

All the yoga nutritional therapy recommendations bring an energetic and biochemical balance to the stomach by providing a proper mix of soothing and tonifying vitamins and phytochemicals.

DIET

Any agent that can irritate the mucus and inner layers of the stomach and duodenum (upper part of the small intestine) must be eradicated from the diet. In a severe case of ulcers, whole grains, nuts, and whole-grain breads and cereals should also be kept away from the diet in the first part of the treatment. All sour fruits, citrus fruits, and fried foods must be limited as well. Alarm foods such as coffee, alcohol, tobacco, tea, salt, and all strong spices should not be part of your diet if ulcers are a concern. Consume all meals and drinks at room temperature or body temperature. Avoid consuming drinks and food that are either too cold or too hot.

For duodenal ulcers, I suggest drinking raw, fresh cabbage juice several times a day. For taste, mix half and half with carrot or celery juice. Raw potato juice is also exceptionally helpful for the treatment of duodenal ulcers.

For stomach ulcers, raw, fresh potato juice with a small amount of cabbage juice three times a day on an empty stomach is very good.

Both cabbage juice and potato juice must be consumed immediately after being prepared, before they lose their medicinal value. Also, eat plenty of dark, green leafy vegetables, and if symptoms are severe, eat soft foods such as squash, bananas, avocados, potatoes, and yams.

SUPPLEMENTS AND SPECIFIC NUTRIENTS

Primary

Everyone should take a high potency multiple vitamin and mineral supplement, as explained in the fifth principle (see page 120). In addition, for the treatment of excess stomach acid and ulcers, I recommend taking the following nutrients:

Vitamin E: 800 IU per day. Deficiency of vitamin E has been linked with intestinal cancer.

Vitamin A: 25,000 to 40,000 units per day. Vitamin A protects the mucus membranes and helps with healing.

Secondary

Brewer's yeast: 2 to 3 tablespoons per day. Brewer's yeast is rich in B vitamins, which balance gastric juices in the stomach.

HERBS

Primary

Aloe vera Juice: 1 or 2 ounces per day to help with pain and accelerates healing.

Turmeric: One 250-mg capsule three times per day or added to food. Turmeric has an anti-inflammatory effect that protects the cell lining of the gastrointestinal tract.

LIVER

The liver is one of the most important organs in the body. Many people develop an enlarged liver, and the main cause is excessive toxicity in the system over the lifetime. The liver's function is to filter toxins from the blood. If the liver is overtaxed by a super abundance of toxins, its function can be reduced.

Among the many factors that affect the liver are extensive use of medications; alcohol intake; meat; heavy, greasy, processed foods; eggs; chemical exposure; and pollution.

Diet

Consuming a proper diet is the only way to cleanse the liver. The best foods to help detoxify the liver are horseradish, red radishes, daikon radish, artichokes, beets and beet greens, onions, carrots, green vegetables, oranges, watermelon, and mangoes.

A very simple recipe for treating liver problems is to steam beets, peel and mash them, then add a little Braggs Liquid Aminos and the seeds of one or two cardamom pods per person. This preparation will act as a total liver rejuvenation treatment. If you have a healthy lifestyle and eat this three days a month, it will also help prevent any future liver problems.

SUPPLEMENTS AND SPECIFIC NUTRIENTS

Primary

Everyone should take a high-potency multiple vitamin and mineral supplement, as explained in the fifth principle (see page 120), along with the following nutrients to attain optimal liver function:

Longevity Green Drink (see Appendix E, Resources) or other green powder: ½ to 1 scoop once or twice per day is extremely beneficial if you have liver disease. Longevity Green Drink will bring trace elements and oxygen into your blood, and this will help detoxify the liver.

Secondary
Alpha-lipoic acid: 100 mg two times per day. Alpha-lipoic acid is a powerful antioxidant and helps protect the liver from alcohol damage.

Evening primrose oil: 1,000 mg three times per day provides essential fatty acids necessary for the rebuilding of liver function.

Pycnogenol: 30 mg three times per day. Pycnogenol is a powerful antioxidant that protects liver cells.

HERBS

Primary
Milk thistle: 300 to 800 mg per day, in three divided doses. Milk thistle helps detoxify the liver.

Secondary
Boswellia: 150 mg three times per day. Boswellia is a powerful anti-inflammatory agent and is effective as a yoga nutritional therapy for the liver in this dose.

COLON (INFLAMMATION, CONSTIPATION, AND HEMORRHOIDS)

The last part of the gastrointestinal system is the colon. After nutrients are partially digested in the stomach and assimilated in the small intestine, they pass to the large intestine. In the large intestine, water is added, and the waste products of metabolism are finally eliminated.

DIET

Proper water intake is crucial to colon health. Do you know how much water you drink each day? If not, it's time for you to pay attention to your total water intake. I recommend that you drink 8 to 10 8-ounce glasses of water per day. The water should be at room temperature or lukewarm. Avoid ice water.

For ulcerative colitis, eat more yogurt and onions. Simply add them to your diet.

For an inflamed or irritated colon, eat three bananas followed by the contents of one cardamom pod, once per day, besides your regular meals. You may repeat this until symptoms subside, usually in about three to five days.

For a prolapsed transverse colon, take or drink acidophilus.

For the prevention and relief of constipation, eat apples, bananas, grapes, melons, papaya, dates, black pepper with steamed green vegetables, boiled onions, rye, psyllium, and vegetable broth with potatoes. Incorporate these foods into your diet as much as possible.

For the prevention of diverticulitis, Eat green chilies.

For hemorrhoids, eat beets and beet greens. Hemorrhoids occur when the liver is not working properly. Beets will help cleanse the liver and, in turn, help relieve hemorrhoids. A good topical remedy is to put a few drops of eucalyptus oil in a little warm water and apply to the area to relieve discomfort.

SUPPLEMENTS AND SPECIFIC NUTRIENTS
Primary
Everyone should take a high-potency multiple vitamin and mineral supplement, as explained in the fifth principle (see page 120), plus the following nutrients for colon health:

Longevity Green Drink (see Appendix E, Resources) or other green powder: ½ to 1 scoop in the morning in juice helps eliminate toxins.

Flaxseed oil: 2 teaspoons per day to restore fatty acid balance and aid in proper bowel movement.

Acidophilus: 1 or 2 capsules per day to help normalize bowel function.

Digestive enzymes: 1 to 3 capsules per day to aid digestion and therefore help with intestinal health.

Secondary
Bifidus: 1 to 2 capsules per day to replace bowel flora and improve assimilation of nutrients from foods.

HERBS
Primary
Aloe vera juice: Drink ½ cup in the morning and ½ cup in the evening. Aloe vera helps heal and cleanse the intestinal tract.

Secondary
Aloe vera bark: 450 mg in capsules. Take one as needed for constipation.

Milk thistle: 300 to 800 mg per day to help detoxify the liver and ease bowel movements.

Ginger: 500 mg twice per day. Drink in tea or take in capsule form. Stimulates digestion and intestinal health.

JUICE

Digestive Soother
Makes 1 serving

2 medium carrots
3 celery stalks
½ cucumber

Juice all ingredients and enjoy. Digestive soother is beneficial to the health of the entire digestive system. Use it to treat any digestive condition. Fresh juices are best consumed within 2 or 3 hours of preparation and should be refrigerated.

RECIPE

Baked Pears
Makes 4 servings

3 large dates, finely chopped
½ cup granola
1 tablespoon ground flaxseeds
¼ teaspoon cinnamon
¼ teaspoon fresh ginger, grated
1 tablespoon apple juice
4 medium pears, peeled and cored
1 cup apple juice

In a mixing bowl, combine dates, granola, flaxseeds, cinnamon, ginger, and 1 tablespoon apple juice. Carefully core pears, then fill them with the granola mix. Place them in a baking pan, then add 1 cup apple juice to prevent sticking. Bake at 350°F for 35 minutes. Check after 15 minutes, and ladle juice over the pears so they won't darken or dry on the outside. Pears are easily digested and are very calming for the whole digestive system.

CHAPTER 29

Heart Disease, Hypertension, and High Cholesterol

HEART DISEASE

Heart disease is America's number one killer. Nearly 62 million people in the United States have some form of cardiovascular disease. At least one million Americans die of the disease every year. According to the American Heart Association, about one third of those deaths could be prevented by better eating practices. Conventional treatment, however, uses drugs and surgery to treat heart disease, with a slight emphasis on prevention via dietary change and exercise.

John Goodman, the author of *Cardiovascular Megatrends: The 21st Century,* has called heart surgery "the most exploding field in health care." Each year, he says, about 1.4 million Americans have either coronary bypass surgery or angioplasty. The American Heart Association reports that the hospital care, doctors' bills, and drug costs of caring for patients with heart disease add up to $115 billion annually.

As a rapidly growing body of evidence suggests, heart disease is a disease of inflammation. We have come to appreciate in recent years that this inflammation can explain why people with no known risk factors such as high cholesterol or high blood pressure can still have heart attacks. Inflammation damages the walls of arteries, making them more prone to fatty buildup. Moreover, weight gain around the abdominal area triggers an inflammatory response and significantly elevates the risk of heart disease, especially in women. There is also evidence that common infections such as cold sores, upper respiratory infections, and genital herpes are significantly linked to the development of heart disease via the inflammatory process.

Additionally, heart disease is directly related to several other conditions, such as arteriosclerosis, circulatory problems, hypertension, and high cholesterol. All these conditions can be substantially prevented or reversed by following the prescription outlined below for heart disease.

DIET

What can you do to avoid heart disease? Follow the yoga nutritional therapy anti-inflammatory diet. If you have heart disease, following a yoga nutritional therapy dietary program can help you avoid surgery.

For phytonutrients, eat fresh fruit and raw vegetables. Among the many sources of dietary fiber, such as cereal, vegetables, and fruits, the oat fiber found in oatmeal and other breakfast cereals appears to be the most beneficial. Add garlic and onions to your diet, since they contain compounds that help reduce serum cholesterol levels. Eat raw nuts (except peanuts), extra virgin olive oil, pink salmon, tuna, and Atlantic herring. These foods contain essential fatty acids. Stay away from all sources of sodium and from food products that have salt, soda, sodium, or the symbol Na on the label.

If you are considered at risk for a heart attack, follow these yoga nutritional therapy principles:

- Make sure your diet is rich in fiber.
- Eat foods rich in vitamins B_6 and B_{12}, which occur naturally in leafy green vegetables and fruits.
- Folic acid prevents heart disease and can be found in cereals, asparagus, spinach, chickpeas, and beans. Include almonds, brewer's yeast, grains, and sesame seeds in your diet as well. They are all high in folic acid.
- Do not eat red meat, salt, sugar, or white flour.
- Eat soy-based protein foods, which can effectively lower high LDL cholesterol levels.
- Eliminate fried foods from your diet, and reduce coffee, black tea, colas, and other alarm food stimulants.
- Do not smoke, and avoid secondhand smoke.
- Eat avocados. Their oil is similar to olive oil and helps lower cholesterol levels.

- Eat apples. Apples contain pectin, a soluble fiber that melts LDL cholesterol.
- Use the anti-inflammatory spices turmeric, ginger, cumin, and cloves.
- Avoid margarine, shortening, and processed oils such as cottonseed oil.

SPECIAL FOODS FOR HEART DISEASE

Brazil nuts, puffed wheat, and oat bran contain vitamin E and selenium. Vitamin E is a powerful antioxidant, and selenium is an important nutrient for optimal heart muscle function.

Dark orange and dark leafy green vegetables, such as sweet potatoes, carrots, pumpkin, dried apricots, collards, spinach, and kale are all rich in carotenoids. These potent anti-inflammatory molecules protect your arteries.

Asparagus, watermelon, strawberries, and fresh peaches all contain the powerful antioxidant glutathione, which retards inflammation while helping your genes send a positive healing message to your heart.

SUPPLEMENTS AND SPECIFIC NUTRIENTS

Primary

Everyone should take a high-potency multiple vitamin and mineral supplement, as explained in the fifth principle (see page 120). To prevent or help heart disease, I also recommend the following nutrients:

Vitamin E: 600 to 1,200 IU per day for prevention. Vitamin E is an efficient antioxidant that increases blood flow and helps reduce the risk of heart attack.

Coenzyme Q10: 100 to 300 mg per day. Coenzyme Q10 boosts oxygenation to the heart muscle.

Grapeseed extract: 150 to 300 mg per day. Grapeseed extract strengthens the cardiovascular system.

Essential fatty acids: 20 to 40 grams of EFAs per day in the form of Borage oil, fish oil, evening primrose oil, or flax oil. Essential fatty acids reduce cholesterol and fat in the blood.

Secondary
Alpha-lipoic acid: 250 to 500 mg per day. Alpha lipoic acid helps lower LDL or bad cholesterol.

DHEA AND HEART DISEASE

Dehydroepiandrosterone (DHEA) is a hormone that is secreted by the adrenal glands. It is active in virtually every cell of the body. As we age, DHEA levels in the blood tend to decrease; this decrease has been shown to be detrimental to heart health. According to a significant study in the *American Journal of Epidemiology* in 2001, low levels of DHEA are associated with higher levels of heart disease in middle-aged men. Over 1,709 men aged 40 to 70 years were tested; the results showed that those with the lowest levels of DHEA were more likely to develop heart disease. This result was independent of other risk factors such as age, obesity, diabetes, hypertension, smoking, serum lipids, alcohol intake, and physical activity.

I suggest that every person over forty-five have his or her blood DHEA measured and then replaced to the level of a thirty-year-old. The typical dose I use is 25 to 100 mg per day. Men need to have a prostate test before starting DHEA and take a saw palmetto formula along with it, because of the theoretical concern that DHEA may be associated with prostate enlargement.

HERBS

Secondary
Hawthorn berries: 2 to 4 standardized tablets per day. Hawthorn berries are a cardiovascular tonic. There are no contraindications, but the herb has not been studied in patients who are taking cardiovascular drugs. Therefore, use it under the care of a knowledgeable herbalist or health care practitioner.

Gingko biloba: 120 mg per day. Ginkgo is a powerful antioxidant and circulation enhancer. It inhibits platelet aggregation, which lessens the chance of a blood clot forming in an artery.

HYPERTENSION

Blood pressure can be defined as the pressure or force that is applied against the artery walls as blood is carried through the circulatory system. It is recorded as a measurement of this force in relation to the heart's pumping activity, and is measured in millimeters of mercury. In people with hypertension, this pressure is abnormally high. Whether blood pressure is high, low, or normal depends on several factors: the output from the heart, the resistance to blood flow of the blood vessels, the volume of blood, and the distribution of blood to the various organs. If blood pressure is high, the heart must work harder to pump adequate amounts of blood to all the tissues of the body. High blood pressure can lead to coronary heart disease, arteriosclerosis, strokes, and kidney failure. It kills 45,000 Americans outright and contributes to the deaths of an additional 210,000 people each year.

A staggering study published in the *Journal of the American Medical Association* in March 2002 predicted that nine of ten middle-aged Americans will, at some point, develop high blood pressure. The American Heart Association, which urged all Americans to prevent this disease by following what in essence is a yoga nutritional therapy diet, considered this study a wake-up call. Beyond that, Claude Lenfant, the director of the National Heart, Lung and Blood Institute in Bethesda, Maryland, has said, "Lifestyle changes can have a big impact, and it's never too late to start."

Because high blood pressure usually causes no symptoms until complications develop, it is known as the silent killer. Warning signs associated with high blood pressure are headaches, sweating, rapid pulse, shortness of breath, dizziness, and visual disturbances.

DIET

To lower blood pressure, follow a strict salt-free diet. Read labels carefully, and avoid food products that have salt, soda, sodium, or the symbol Na on the label. Other foods and food additives that should be avoided are baking soda, canned vegetables (unless marked sodium- or salt-free), diet soft drinks, foods with mold inhibitors, preservatives and/or sugar substitutes, softened water, and soy sauce.

Bacon, beef, bouillons, liver, corned beef, dairy products, gravies, pork, sausage, and smoked or processed meats are prohibited. Avoid high-saturated-fat alarm foods such as aged cheeses and aged meats, as well as anchovies (because of their salt content), and sugar-laden chocolate. These foods contribute to hardening of the arteries, which causes narrowing of the blood vessels, leading to high blood pressure. Avoid all alcohol, caffeine, and tobacco.

What can you eat to lower your blood pressure? That's easy. Eat lots of fresh fruits and vegetables, such as apples, asparagus, bananas, broccoli, cabbage, cantaloupe, eggplant, garlic, grapefruit, green leafy vegetables, melons, peas, prunes, raisins, squash, and sweet potatoes. Eat grains such as quinoa (keen-wa), brown rice, buckwheat, millet, and oats. Eat broiled white fish, salmon, and skinless turkey or chicken, in moderation.

Another consideration in keeping your blood pressure under control is to keep your weight down. If you are overweight, take steps to lose the excess pounds. Healthful ways to do that include fasting three to five days each month, getting regular exercise, and meditating to reduce the effects of stress. Be sure to get sufficient sleep.

SUPPLEMENTS AND SPECIFIC NUTRIENTS

Primary

Everyone should take a high-potency multiple vitamin and mineral supplement, as explained in the fifth principle (see page 120). This basic supplement contains all the important antihypertension minerals. In addition, I recommend taking the following nutrients to help stabilize hypertension:

Coenzyme Q10: 100 to 300 mg per day. Coenzyme Q10 increases oxygenation by boosting blood flow.

Secondary

Vitamin C: 3,000 to 6,000 mg per day in divided doses. Vitamin C is essential in regulating high blood pressure.

HERBS

Primary

Garlic: Garlic is best taken by adding it to your food. You can also take a deodorized form in the amount of 5 to 10 mg per day. Garlic prevents the deposition of fats in the arteries.

HIGH CHOLESTEROL

High cholesterol is associated with a greater than normal risk of arteriosclerosis and cardiovascular disease. Knowing and controlling your cholesterol levels is a very important step in preventing these diseases. There are different types of cholesterol, and they have different functions.

Low-density lipoprotein (LDL) is known as the bad cholesterol. It carries most of the cholesterol in the blood and is the main source of damaging accumulation and blockage in the arteries.

High-density lipoprotein (HDL) is known as the good cholesterol. It transports cholesterol from the blood back to the liver, where it is eliminated from the body. HDL cholesterol also can help keep LDL cholesterol from building up in the walls of the arteries.

Triglycerides are a form of fat carried in the bloodstream. The body's most abundant fat is in the form of triglycerides, which are stored in fat tissue. A smaller amount of tryglycerides is found in the bloodstream. High levels of triglycerides in the bloodstream also contribute to coronary heart disease.

The safe level of cholesterol in the blood, set by the National Cholesterol Education Program, is less than 200 milligrams per deciliter of blood. This includes both LDL and HDL. If you have a cholesterol reading below 180, with HDL at 80 and LDL at 120, you are considered at a low risk for heart disease. If your levels are above 200 for cholesterol, with HDL below 45 and LDL above 150, your risk is elevated, and you need to be under the care of a nutritionally oriented physician.

THE DRUG TREATMENT OF HIGH CHOLESTEROL

Many people with high cholesterol are being treated with drugs called statins. Six statins are now on the market in the United States, and about 12 million people take them. These medications were initially thought to be life saving and free of side effects, but they're not. In fact, on August 8, 2001, one of them, Baycol, was taken off the market after 31 patients died. The deaths were caused by a disorder in which muscle cells break down, overwhelming the kidneys with cellular waste three months earlier.

Unfortunately, this recall followed a push three months earlier by drug companies and the federal government to expand the use of statins to 36 million Americans. The problems associated with statins, which in addition to the muscle disease cited above include liver damage, raise many questions about how doctors approach the treatment of heart disease in general and elevated cholesterol levels in particular.

Many experts who practice alternative approaches to the treatment of heart disease believe that cholesterol drugs do almost nothing to eliminate the risk of a heart attack, except in rare cases. But I believe statins have a role in modern medicine. I also know that a yoga nutritional therapy approach can help you reduce your cholesterol level and promote heart health, whether you take statins or not. Beyond that, if you do take statin drugs, realize that they deplete your heart muscle of coenzyme Q10. Therefore, you must take coenzyme Q10 in a dose of 100 to 300 mg per day if you take statin drugs or if you have significant heart disease.

DIET

Saturated fat, found mostly in foods that come from animals, increases your LDL cholesterol level more than anything else in your diet. Reducing the amount of saturated fat and LDL cholesterol in your diet is a very significant step toward reducing cholesterol levels. Cholesterol is found in red meat, poultry, seafood, and dairy products. You'll want to limit these foods in your diet.

I recommend eliminating all hydrogenated and hardened fats and oils such as margarine, lard, and butter. Do not consume heated fats, processed oils, hard liquor, cakes, candy, carbonated drinks, coffee, gravies, nondairy creamers, pies, processed or refined foods, tobacco, or white bread. Avoid pork and pork products.

Apples, bananas, grapefruit, carrots, dried beans, garlic, oat bran, and olive oil are cholesterol-lowering foods. Make them a large part of your diet. Also, fruits, vegetables, vegetable oils, grains, cereals, nuts, and seeds do not contain cholesterol.

SUPPLEMENTS AND SPECIFIC NUTRIENTS

Primary

Everyone should take a high-potency multiple vitamin and mineral supplement, as explained in the fifth principle (see page 120). In addition, to help lower cholesterol, I suggest taking the following supplements:

Coenzyme Q10: 100 to 3,000 mg per day to strengthen the cardiac muscle.

Vitamin C: 3,000 to 8,000 mg per day to help lower cholesterol.

Vitamin E: 400 to 800 IU per day. This amount is often found in a multiple vitamin formula. Vitamin E improves the circulation.

Chromium picolinate: 200 mcg per day. This amount should be in the daily multiple vitamin and mineral supplement you are already taking. Chromium helps regulate insulin levels, which control fat deposition in your arteries.

Secondary
Inositol hexaniacinate (IN): 1,000 to 1,500 mg per day in three divided doses is excellent for lowering cholesterol, especially when used together with gugulipids, as described below. IN is a form of the B vitamin niacin but does not have its annoying side effects, such as flushing and blushing.

HERBS

Primary
Gugulipid: 175 mg three times per day, at a minimum. Gugulipid is an extract from the mukul tree that has had a long illustrious history in yoga nutritional therapy. Clinical evidence shows that it lowers cholesterol and triglyerides levels by up to 30 percent by supporting the liver in processing cholesterol. Gugulipid is best taken in conjunction with inositol hexaniacinate, chromium picolinate, guar gum, and artichoke extract. *Note:* Because gugulipid may affect the platelets, please discuss its use with your doctor if you are taking blood thinners.

Secondary
Artichoke extract: 150 mg per day works in synergy with the other nutrients to control cholesterol by affecting its metabolism.
Hawthorn berries: 2 to 4 standardized tablets per day to help lower cholesterol.
Guar gum: 225 mg per day to help control cholesterol by increasing its elimination.

JUICE

To combat heart disease, hypertension, and high cholesterol levels, drink fresh juices, especially carrot, celery, and beet juices. Carrot juice helps flush out fat from the bile in the liver, and this helps lower cholesterol.

Anticholesterol Juice
Makes 1 serving

> handful parsley
> handful spinach
> 2 carrots, greens removed
> 1 garlic clove

Wash and dry the parsley, spinach, and carrots. Peel the garlic, and juice with remaining ingredients. Fresh juices are best consumed within 2 to 3 hours of preparation and should be refrigerated.

RECIPE

Nirvair's Baked Tofu with Salad
Makes 4 servings

This recipe is good for lowering your risk of heart disease, hypertension, and high cholesterol.

1 block firm tofu, approximately 16 ounces
½ teaspoon extra virgin olive oil
juice of 1 lemon
¼ cup Braggs Liquid Aminos

SALAD:
4 cups mixed baby greens
2 scallions, chopped
½ red bell pepper, sliced medium thin
1 tomato, diced
½ cucumber, peeled and sliced
1 carrot, grated

HONEY MUSTARD DRESSING:
¼ teaspoon minced garlic
2 tablespoons apple cider vinegar
¼ cup unsweetened apple juice
1 tablespoon plus 1 teaspoon honey
2 teaspoons Dijon mustard
1 tablespoon extra virgin olive oil

Preheat the oven to 400°F. Unpack tofu and drain off excess water. Wrap tofu in a paper towel and let sit for 5 to 10 minutes to absorb any extra water. Cut the tofu lengthwise into three slices, then cut each slice in half. You will have a total of six slices. Place tofu slices into a lightly oiled baking pan. Pour half the lemon juice over the tofu, sprinkle with half the Braggs Liquid Aminos, and bake for approximately 20 minutes. Turn the tofu slices over, sprinkle with the rest of the lemon juice and Braggs Liquid Aminos, and bake for another 20 minutes, until slightly crisp. You can vary the cooking times—less for softer tofu, more for crispier tofu.

In the meantime, prepare your salad dressing by whisking together the garlic, vinegar, juice, honey, and mustard. Slowly pour in the olive oil and whisk together to slightly thicken. Toss the salad, and let sit for about 15 minutes. This will help make it more easily digestible, as the salad dressing will start breaking down the food chemicals.

Divide the salad among four plates. Cut each piece of tofu in half, for a total of twelve slices. Arrange three slices of tofu on each salad.

Tofu, an excellent source of protein and isoflavones without the high fat and artificial hormone content of meat and chicken, is beneficial for all heart conditions.

CHAPTER 30

HIV and AIDS

Infection with the human immunodeficiency virus (HIV) is one of the greatest tragedies of our era. When infection with HIV progresses to serious illness, it is called acquired immunodeficiency syndrome (AIDS). The good news is that people can live with HIV and AIDS if they take very good care of themselves. In strong clinical work performed by my colleague and health psychologist, Shanti Shanti Kaur Khalsa, Ph.D., yoga nutritional therapy has been shown to be very effective in maximizing the health of people with HIV and AIDS.

DIET

Diet is an effective and important component of a program to treat HIV and AIDS. I recommend the mung beans and rice recipe (see page 80), with the trinity roots garlic, onions, and ginger, sautéed in a little ghee, plus lots of fresh ground black pepper. It purifies the blood. Make a mixture of the onions, garlic, and ginger and store it in your refrigerator. Add it to your other meals each day for blood purification.

Drinking six cups or more of Yogi Tea per day (recipe on p. 138) keeps the blood strong and helps cleanse the liver. You can use regular or soy milk, apple juice, or orange juice in the tea. Each morning, after brushing your teeth and before consuming any food or drink, drink a glass of cold Yogi Tea mixed half and half with apple juice. Sip it slowly. This benefits the liver, which must be kept healthy when you have HIV infection or AIDS. A slice or two of daikon radish, steamed or raw, also helps the liver.

For optimal immune system function, be sure to follow all the other yoga nutritional therapy principles.

SUPPLEMENTS AND SPECIFIC NUTRIENTS

Primary

Everyone should take a high-potency multiple vitamin and mineral supplement, as explained in the fifth principle (see page 120). In addition, I recommend that patients with HIV infection or AIDS take the following nutrients:

Vitamin A: 50,000 IU per day for its immune-strengthening and antioxidant effects.

Vitamin C: up to 10 g per day, as tolerated, for its immune-strengthening and antioxidant effects.

Vitamin E: 1,000 IU per day for its immune-strengthening and antioxidant effects.

Coenzyme Q10: 100 mg per day for cellular energy production.

Alpha-lipoic acid: 250 mg per day for cellular energy production.

N-acetylcysteine: 250 mg per day for support of the immune system.

HERBS

Primary

Indian gentian: 5 to 20 mg per kilogram of body weight, or about 340 to 1,000 mg per day. Early clinical trials in HIV-infected men have suggested that Indian gentian extract may lead to a modest improvement in immune function.

Secondary

Turmeric: 100 to 200 mg once or twice per day for its anti-inflammatory properties.

Gingerroot: 500 mg twice per day for its antiviral properties.

Garlic: 4 to 5 mg per day for its antibacterial properties.

MGN3: 3 grams per day. As I discussed in chapter 12 on the fifth principle, MGN3 is a newer product, made from rice bran, that greatly enhances your immune system by increasing the activity of your natural killer cells. It is primarily used to treat cancer and AIDS.

JUICE

Daikon Veggie Kyolic

1 cucumber
4 celery stalks

2 daikons
¾ teaspoon kyolic garlic extract

Wash and dry cucumber, celery, and daikons. Peel the cucumber. Remove the leaves of the celery and cut off the ends. Peel the daikons and cut off the ends. Juice the cucumber, celery, and daikons to make ⅓ cup cucumber juice, ⅓ cup celery juice, and ⅓ cup daikon juice.

Stir the juices together, and strain. There should be 1 cup of juice in total. Add kyolic garlic extract. Drink as soon as possible. Fresh juices are best consumed within 2 to 3 hours of preparation and should be refrigerated.

Cucumber juice soothes the stomach and spleen, is a blood purifier, and helps eliminate phlegm from the lungs. Celery is a natural relaxant, daikon is a powerful liver detoxifying agent, and garlic boosts the immune system and is a blood purifier. Drink this juice once per day.

RECIPES

Jalapeno Immune System Drink

According to yoga nutritional therapy, jalapenos can markedly boost the immune system, thanks to their high content of vitamin C. They help eliminate parasites, improve lung function, stave off colds, and reduce bronchial ailments. Blend raw whole jalapenos with 8 to 12 ounces milk in a Vita-Mix or blender for a couple of minutes. Then sip through a straw. Start with half a jalapeno and gradually work your way up to five jalapenos.

For Blood Cleansing and Antiviral Effects

Combine 1 tablespoon of fresh ground pepper in 1 cup low-fat plain yogurt. Eat at one time or throughout the day. You can build up to 5 tablespoons of pepper over a period of several weeks. This dish may create the feeling of a slight fever for an hour or so as you adjust to its effects.

To Prevent Parasites

Eat one raw onion per day. It can be added to fresh yogurt, salads, steamed vegetables, or rice, as in Mexican food.

Trinity Root Goat's Milk
Makes 1 serving

2 cups goat's milk
½ bulb whole garlic cloves
1″ × 1″ piece gingerroot, peeled & chopped
½ white onion, chopped into small pieces
½ level teaspoon turmeric (*not* rounded, or it will be too
    strong)

Put ingredients in pressure cooker, on medium heat. Slowly heat until hot, and then put lid and pressure valve on securely. When valve begins to release steam and jiggle, cook for exactly 5 minutes, then immediately take pressure cooker off stove and put under cold water for 1 minute. Next, take off pressure valve. If steam is coming out, wait until all steam stops, and only then open the lid. *Note:* If lid is taken off while steam is still coming out, the contents will explode! It is very important to wait. After pressure cooker is cool and has been opened, strain the goat's milk. Discard the onion, garlic, and ginger. Drink this milk while it is still warm, one serving per day.

Milk accelerates the assimilation of the nutrients into the system and tissues. This recipe has antibacterial, antiviral, and anti-inflammatory properties and boosts the immune system.

CHAPTER 31

Immune Health

Your immune system is responsible for seeking out and destroying bacteria and viruses set upon invading your system and making you sick. This is called immune system surveillance. Most people's immune systems break down from chronic, unbalanced stress combined with poor nutrition. Stress depletes the body of vitamin C, B vitamins, and minerals such as magnesium, which keep the immune system strong.

DIET

The yoga nutritional therapy diet is a natural immune system enhancer. In this diet, the primary foods that help boost your immune system are garlic, onions, and ginger. Add onions, garlic, and ginger to the mung beans and rice recipe (see page 80) and to many of your other meals, if possible, for immune system enhancement. All fresh vegetables and fruits are also excellent for the immune system. Also, be sure to eat shiitake, enokidake, maitake, and oyster mushrooms, which are known to strengthen the immune system.

SUPPLEMENTS AND SPECIFIC NUTRIENTS

Primary

Everyone should take a high-potency multiple vitamin and mineral supplement, as explained in the fifth principle (see page 120). In addition, I recommend taking the following nutrients for immune system enhancement:

Vitamin C: 3,000 to 10,000 mg per day. Vitamin C protects against infections.

Secondary
MGN3: 3 grams per day. MGN3 is a newer product, made from rice bran, that greatly enhances your immune system by increasing the activity of your natural killer cells. Although it is primarily used to treat cancer and AIDS, many people take it for immune system support.

HERBS

Primary
Echinacea: 500 to 1,000 mg three times per day. In liquid extract or in capsule form, echinacea is a natural antibiotic. It is particularly effective when used in combination with Vitamin C.

Secondary
Ginseng: 250 to 500 mg per day to boost energy and immunity. Ginseng is particularly effective during recovery from an illness.
Pycnogenol: 100 mg per day to boost the immune system.

JUICE

Antioxidant Plus
Makes 1 serving

½ cup blueberries
1 bunch grapes
½ apple

Wash and dry all ingredients, then juice them. Fresh juices are best consumed within 2 to 3 hours of preparation and should be refrigerated.

Blueberries, grapes, and apples contain very high amounts of nutrients and antioxidants that support immune function.

RECIPE

Boost-Your-Immune-System Breakfast
Makes 1 serving

5 almonds
or
5 pistachios

or

5 cashews

1 to 2 teaspoons fresh ginger, peeled, then grated or chopped
    very fine

½ teaspoon extra virgin olive oil

1 cup low-fat plain yogurt

Sauté the nuts and ginger in olive oil for 3 minutes, then add
the yogurt. Cook well for another 3 to 5 minutes, until mixture becomes brown. Eat as your first meal in the morning.

Almonds, pistachios, and cashews are a source of protein and
omega-3 oils. They help bone marrow, nerves, and reproductive tissues, and they enhance memory and creativity. Ginger is a natural
anti-inflammatory, and yogurt provides protein and accelerates the
absorption of these nutrients by the tissues. This ancient yoga nutritional recipe is recommended to assist the immune system, especially in the prevention of colds, coughs, and the flu.

CHAPTER 32

Kidney Disease

Almost 20 million adult Americans have chronic kidney disease. Normally, the kidneys remove waste from the bloodstream. In chronic disease, they lose their filtering ability, and a person can die without dialysis or a kidney transplant. Kidney disease is among the top ten killers in America. It is a complication of hypertension and diabetes.

Kidney stones are one of the most common kidney problems and one of the most painful conditions—including childbirth—that anyone can have. Ten percent of all Americans will have a kidney stone at some time. Low calcium intake is considered to be a cause of kidney stones. Kidney stones can require surgery and may be life threatening.

Research into the nutritional prevention of kidney stones has revealed the following:

- Dietary calcium from food or supplements reduces the risk of kidney stones.
- Calcium supplementation must be taken with food, in doses of about 400 mg. Getting calcium from a multivitamin is okay as long as it is taken with food.
- A yoga nutritional therapy plant-based diet, which is high in calcium, fiber, vitamins, antioxidants, and plant-based protein, is an excellent way to prevent kidney stones from occurring or recurring.

DIET

Avoid animal protein in your diet, and replace it with vegetable protein, such as soy, whenever possible. Shun vegetables containing large quantities of oxalic acid, such as spinach and rhubarb, as well as caffeine and processed foods.

Follow a yoga nutritional therapy diet, which emphasizes raw and cooked vegetables and raw fruits. Garlic, potatoes, asparagus, parsley, horseradish, cucumber, and celery are excellent vegetables for supporting the kidneys. Fruits that are particularly helpful to the kidneys include papaya, bananas, watermelon, and cranberries; the latter promote healing of the bladder and destroy bacteria buildup, which makes the job of the kidneys easier. Also, increase your consumption of foods rich in vitamin A, such as apricots, cantaloupes, carrots, pumpkins, sweet potatoes, and squash. Finally, drink eight glasses of pure water a day if your kidney function is normal.

SUPPLEMENTS AND SPECIFIC NUTRIENTS

Primary

Everyone should take a high-potency multiple vitamin and mineral supplement, as explained in the fifth principle (see page 120). For optimal kidney function, I also recommend taking the following nutrients:

Vitamin A: 75,000 units per day. After three months, reduce to 10,000 units. Vitamin A helps in the healing of the urinary tract. You should be under your doctor's care when taking high doses of Vitamin A.

Zinc: 50 to 80 mg per day. Do not exceed 100 mg per day. Zinc inhibits crystallization and stimulates healing.

Secondary

Vitamin B complex: 50 mg of each major B vitamin, three times per day. Do not take with milk. Vitamin B helps reduce fluid retention.

HERBS

Secondary

Phyllanthus: 250 to 500 mg three times per day. Phyllantus acts as a detoxifying herb, and no side effects have been reported.

JUICE

Watermelon, cucumber, celery, and cranberry juices all provide a flush to the kidneys. If bladder infections are a problem, a study published in the *British Medical Journal* in June 2001 disclosed that drinking cranberry juice can prevent this common problem, which affects 11.5 million women each year.

Kidney Soother
Makes 1 serving

1-inch slice of ginger
½ cup frozen raspberries
1 cup watermelon, diced
½ cup ice

Wash and dry the ginger, then peel it. Juice the raspberries, watermelon, and ginger. Pour the juice over ice, and drink cold. Fresh juices are best consumed within 2 to 3 hours of preparation and should be refrigerated.

Ginger is a natural anti-inflammatory, and the berries and watermelon help flush the kidneys.

RECIPE

Sat's Spring Salad
Makes 2 servings

2 medium heads yellow endive
1 medium apple, sliced thin
½ cup walnuts, chopped
½ cup watercress leaves
¼ cup blue cheese

DRESSING
1 tablespoon nonfat cottage cheese
1 teaspoon apple cider vinegar
3 teaspoons walnut oil
1 medium clove garlic, crushed
salt and pepper to taste

Carefully remove all the leaves of the endive without breaking them. Wash and dry endive, apple, and watercress. Arrange endive leaves at the bottom of each individual plate in a circle, apple slices in the middle, and watercress over endive. Sprinkle walnuts and blue cheese on top.

Place dressing ingredients in a blender or food processor, and puree. Pour over salad, and serve.

Watercress and endive are powerful cleansers of the intestinal and circulatory systems. They also improve kidney function.

Lung Disease: Asthma and Chronic Obstructive Lung Disease, Including Emphysema and Bronchitis

Asthma is increasing in occurrence and severity in America for a myriad of reasons, including diet and air pollution. According to a 1995 study, mortality rates from asthma doubled in America from 1978 to 1987. What can we do to decrease this statistic? Plenty. Please read on. Because the underlying pathologic changes are the same for asthma, emphysema, and bronchitis, the suggestions below are effective for all of them.

DIET

Epidemiological studies suggest that dietary habits influence lung function in asthma, emphysema, and chronic bronchitis. The imbalance of omega-6 fats, as found in meat, relative to omega-3 fats, as found in fish, is believed to play a significant role in the development of asthma. Foods to reduce in the diet, therefore, include meat, shellfish, and vegetable oils. Although this is somewhat controversial—I suggest that you not give your asthmatic child cow's milk.

Food additives can trigger asthma, too. Watch out for peanuts, MSG, and especially aspartame. Foods to eat more of include fatty fish, flaxseed oil, fish oil, and garlic, onions, fruits, and vegetables, which are rich in phytonutrients and antioxidants.

Patience is needed in treating asthma with nutrition, as reports show that up to one year may be needed to reverse the symptoms. You may be able to speed up your healing time by following a short fast or cleansing program.

SUPPLEMENTS AND SPECIFIC NUTRIENTS

Primary

Everyone should take a high-potency multiple vitamin and mineral supplement, as explained in the fifth principle (see page 120). Children need to take a children's vitamin without any fillers or aspartame. In addition, I recommend the following nutrients to help heal asthma, emphysema, and bronchitis:

Vitamin C: up to 3,000 mg per day, to protect lung tissue.

Coenzyme Q10: 100 mg per day, to fight against histamine, which leads to airway constriction.

Magnesium sulfate: 250 to 1,000 mg per day by your doctor. Magnesium augments the vital capacity of the lungs.

Selenium: 100 mcg per day, to fight against air pollutants.

Secondary

Molybdenum: 1 to 3 mg per day; may improve lung function.

N-*acetylcysteine:* 250 mg per day, to rebuild lung tissue.

Vitamin B$_{12}$: 1,000 mcg per day may also help reduce inflammation in the lungs.

HERBS

Primary

Green tea: 150 mg per day, either in beverage or in supplement form, to help relax the airways. Green tea contains anti-inflammatory phytonutrients, which decrease lung inflammation. It also has a mild bronchodilating effect.

JUICE
Antioxidant Boost
Makes 1 serving

> 2 large carrots
> 1 celery stalk
> 2 leaves and stems of beet greens
> dash of Tabasco

Wash and dry the carrots, celery, and beet greens, then juice them. Add Tabasco, and enjoy. Fresh juices are best consumed within 2 to 3 hours of preparation and should be refrigerated.

The antioxidant boost recipe provides high amounts of minerals and antioxidants that support optimal lung function.

RECIPE

Quinoa Salad
Makes 4 servings

1 cup dry quinoa (keen-wa)
2 cups water
1½ cups chopped organic broccoli crowns
½ cucumber, peeled, seeded, and finely chopped
¼ cup red onion, finely chopped
1 scallion, including green part, finely chopped
1 medium carrot, grated

DRESSING
¼ cup flaxseed oil
¼ cup lemon juice
1 tablespoon Dijon mustard
½ teaspoon garlic
2 teaspoons zattar (herb mix from Middle Eastern stores)
2 teaspoons honey

Rinse the quinoa in a fine strainer, and allow to drain. Place quinoa and water in a medium saucepan, and bring to a boil (approximately 5 minutes). Then simmer for 20 minutes. Allow to cool in the refrigerator, stirring occasionally. Lightly steam the broccoli, and cool in the refrigerator. Combine the remaining ingredients with the cooled quinoa and broccoli. In a separate bowl, whisk dressing ingredients together. Drizzle dressing over quinoa salad and serve.

This salad provides high amounts of minerals and antioxidants that support optimal lung function, plus high-quality protein in the easy-to-digest quinoa.

CHAPTER 34

Men's Health: Impotence and Prostate Problems

IMPOTENCE

It is estimated that about 30 million American men are impotent. The causes include prostate enlargement or cancer, psychological issues, aging, and underlying physical illness. Following a yoga nutritional therapy program will not only treat impotence successfully but prevent it as well.

DIET

Elevated alcohol consumption, smoking, high cholesterol, high blood pressure, and diabetes can be contributing factors to impotence. The most commonly prescribed yoga nutritional therapy foods to cure impotence are onions, ginger, garlic, pistachio nuts, almonds, figs, and the spice saffron.

SUPPLEMENTS AND SPECIFIC NUTRIENTS

Primary

Everybody should take a high-potency multiple vitamin and mineral supplement, as explained in the fifth principle (see page 120). In addition, to treat impotence, I recommend taking the following nutrients:

Essential fatty acids: 1,000 mg per day, to support maximum function.

Vitamin C: 1,000 to 5,000 mg per day, to boost the immune system.

Zinc: 80 mg per day is vital to prostate health.

Quercetin: 1,000 to 2,000 mg per day is a natural anti-inflammatory for the prostate.

TESTOSTERONE

Some compounds on the market, usually available at specialty shops rather than regular health food stores, are touted to release testosterone. These formulas are also available without a prescription through a compounding pharmacist. These so-called stacking formulas contain a combination of ingredients that are said to release a man's own testosterone, thus leading to restored sexual vigor, increased muscle mass, greater grip strength, higher energy levels, improved mood, and enhanced memory.

Hormone precursors such as Tribulus Terrestris, for instance, are thought to work by producing more leutinizing hormone, which signals the body to make more testosterone. Some of these formulas also contain another compound, chrysin, which inhibits the conversion of testosterone into estrogen, helping maximize the effects of testosterone while modulating the effects of estrogen in men. Some of the formulas also contain DHEA, which I prefer to administer separately.

You may also find a formula that contains androstenedione as well as 5-androstenediol, two potent male hormones that recent research suggests have their own direct effects, as well as increasing testosterone levels.

I have no doubt these compounds work, but I think they are too extreme to take on a regular basis. If a man is low on testosterone and needs an energy boost for an athletic event or for sexual activity, I think it is acceptable to take a stacking formula under the care of a knowledgeable physician who specializes in anti-aging. For regular use, however, as in hormone replacement therapy, it's my opinion that you should take testosterone by cream, which is rubbed on the skin. Again, please do this only under the care of a knowledgeable doctor.

For more information on testosterone, turn to page 175.

HERBS

Primary

Saw palmetto: 100 to 300 mg per day reduces prostate enlargement by balancing male hormones.

Pygeum: 100 to 200 mg per day helps with urinary problems associated with prostate enlargement.

Lycopene: As little as 4 mg per day will suffice if used in a combination formula such as ProstaCol by Vitamin Research Products (see Appendix E, Resources). If lycopene is taken separately, the dose can go as high as 100 mg per day. Lycopene is also beneficial in preventing prostate enlargement and cancer.

Stinging nettle: 300 mg per day contributes to overall prostate health.

Secondary
Ginseng: 150 to 300 mg per day. Ginseng is an herb beneficial to male energy.

PROSTATE PROBLEMS

Prostate enlargement is common in men as they age.

DIET

You can make some dietary modifications to prevent prostate enlargement or reduce the swelling. First, reduce your fat intake, especially from animal sources, and reduce your intake of saturated fat. Second, eliminate caffeine, alcohol, and black pepper from your diet for optimal prostate health. These substances exacerbate the symptoms of an enlarged prostate.

Soy foods are very beneficial to prostate health, and so are fresh fruits and vegetables. Tomatoes are particularly helpful, especially when cooked. So eat lots of pasta sauce—it's very good for you. Also, whole grains supply essential fatty acids, and sunflower and pumpkin seeds provide zinc, essential for a healthy prostate.

SUPPLEMENTS AND SPECIFIC NUTRIENTS

Primary
Everyone should take a high-potency multiple vitamin and mineral supplement, as explained in the fifth principle (see page 120). In addition, for maximum prostate health, I suggest taking the following nutrients:

Essential fatty acids: 1,000 mg per day for prostate function.

Zinc: 80 mg per day for prostate health.

HERBS

Primary

Saw palmetto: 100 to 300 mg per day reduces prostate enlargement by balancing male hormones.

Pygeum: 100 to 200 mg per day helps with urinary problems associated with prostate enlargement.

Lycopene: As little as 4 mg per day will suffice if used in a combination formula such as ProstaCol by Vitamin Research Products (see Appendix E, Resources). If lycopene is taken separately, the dose can go as high as 100 mg per day. Lycopene is also beneficial in preventing cancer.

Stinging nettle: 300 mg per day contributes to overall prostate health.

Secondary

Ginseng: 150 to 300 mg per day. Ginseng is a male energy herb.

JUICE

Zinc Boost

Makes 1 serving

½-inch slice ginger
3 carrots
½ apple

Wash and dry all ingredients. Peel the ginger, and juice with remaining ingredients. Drink as your midmorning or midafternoon snack. Fresh juices are best consumed within 2 to 3 hours of preparation and should be refrigerated.

Zinc boost helps both impotence and enlarged prostate by boosting the immune system.

RECIPES

Golden Figs

This is a great yoga nutritional therapy recipe for promoting male vitality, potency, strength, and healthy prostate function. Soak four or five stems of saffron in a little milk overnight. In the morning, take a sterile syringe, draw the golden milk, and inject it into some fresh, ripe figs. Enjoy three of them per day, and you will rapidly notice a great difference in energy. The figs can be prepared ahead of time and kept in the freezer for a few days.

Nutty Fruit Salad
Makes 3 servings

2 tablespoons pistachios
2 tablespoons sunflower seeds
2 tablespoons pecans
2 tablespoons pumpkin seeds
1 plum, pitted and chopped
1 peach, pitted, peeled, and chopped
¼ cup pineapple, chopped
½ small papaya, seeded and chopped
2 fresh figs, cut into quarters
juice of 1 lime

Roast the nuts before mixing with the fruit to enhance their flavor. Place nuts on a baking sheet in a 300°F oven for 5 minutes. Check the nuts after 2 minutes because they can burn easily. In a serving bowl, combine the nuts and chopped fruit. Stir in lime juice, toss and serve.

Nuts provide omega-3 oils, zinc, and high-quality protein. The fruits are an important source of minerals and antioxidants, which boost your immune system.

Skin Disorders: Acne and Aging

ACNE

Acne is an inflammatory disease that occurs most commonly during adolescence. Although hormone changes are suspected, the exact cause of
acne is unknown. In my experience, however, diet and chronic, unbalanced
stress clearly affect your skin. A diet high in fat, processed foods, oil, and
sugar presents the body with a heavy toxic load. These toxins must exit the
body somewhere. In people with acne, the toxins are excreted by the skin.

DIET

Research has revealed that people with acne who follow a yoga nutritional
therapy diet show substantial improvement. I suggest beginning with a
short, detoxifying fast. For instructions on fasting, please see page 70. To
break the fast, follow the mung beans and rice recipe (see page 80) for two
to three days. Then, as you begin to incorporate a wide variety of foods into
your yoga nutritional therapy diet, keep in mind that anti-inflammatory oils,
such as those found in cold-water fish, nuts, and seeds, are especially good
for healing acne, as are carotene-rich orange, yellow, and leafy green vegetables. Emphasize raw, fresh fruits and vegetables, and drink at least eight
glasses of pure water per day.

Avoid animal protein as much as possible, and eliminate all sweets and
processed foods—that means no soft drinks, candy, ice cream, or anything
else made with sugar or white flour.

Supplements and Specific Nutrients

Primary

Everyone should take a high-potency multiple vitamin and mineral supplement, as explained in the fifth principle (see page 120). In addition, I recommend taking the following nutrients to help heal your acne:

Vitamin A: Up to 300,000 IU per day, under a doctor's supervision. Vitamin A protects the skin.

Secondary

Evening primrose oil: 500 mg one to three times per day. Primrose oil improves the skin.

Zinc: 50 mg per day. Zinc contributes to tissue healing.

HERBS

Secondary

Milk thistle: 100 to 300 mg per day. Milk thistle helps cleanse your system by detoxifying the liver.

Turmeric: Mix ½ teaspoon of turmeric powder with a few drops of water until you have a paste. Apply to acne lesions and leave on until completely dry, then wash off with warm water. Repeat four times per day. Also, you can add more turmeric to your mung beans and rice recipe (see page 79).

AGING

Free radical damage is considered to be the primary cause of skin aging. Sun exposure, especially during the middle of the day; smoking; a diet rich in red meat; and stress will cause premature aging of the skin by increasing free radical damage. To prevent skin aging, always use sunscreen and limit your sun exposure to the first part of the morning or the latter part of the afternoon.

DIET

The yoga nutritional therapy diet will keep your skin young. It is rich in enzymes, which help with skin repair and cell renewal. It is also rich in foods high in RNA, such as salmon, tuna, lentils, and mung beans. RNA helps improve cell energy, thereby increasing cell renewal in aging skin.

To protect your skin from free radical damage, eat plenty of phytonutrient-rich foods such as fruit, vegetables, and green tea. You will find these foods in abundant supply in the yoga nutritional therapy diet.

SUPPLEMENTS AND SPECIFIC NUTRIENTS

Primary

Everyone should take a high-potency multiple vitamin and mineral supplement, as explained in the fifth principle (see page 120). This supplement contains antioxidant vitamins and the minerals selenium, zinc, copper, and manganese, all of which protect and revitalize your skin. In addition, I recommend the following nutrients to heal aging skin:

Flaxseed oil: 6,000 to 7,000 mg per day. You can also simply add flaxseed oil to your salads and smoothies.

or

Fish oil: 3,000 to 4,000 mg per day. Please note that flaxseed oil is usually easier on your stomach than fish oil.

Secondary

Alpha-lipoic acid: 250 to 500 mg per day, for powerful antioxidant effects.

DHEA and melatonin: A study published in the *Journal of Surgical Research* in October 2001 demonstrated that the hormones DHEA and melatonin, topically applied, are active in skin health and cancer prevention. As their exact roles in human skin are still under scrutiny, this therapy should be undertaken only with the guidance of your health professional.

HERBS

Primary

Milk thistle: 100 to 300 mg per day to help detoxify the tissues.

JUICE

Skin Rejuvenator for Acne and Aging
Makes 1 serving

2 medium carrots
1 celery stalk

½ cucumber
¼ to ½ golden delicious apple for sweetness

Wash and dry all the ingredients. Peel the cucumber, and juice with remaining ingredients. Fresh juices are best consumed within 2 to 3 hours of preparation and should be refrigerated.

Cucumber juice is a blood purifier and relieves acne. Celery and carrots provide nutrients that maintain youthful-looking skin.

RECIPE

Rudy's Summer Salad
Makes 4 servings

1 cucumber, peeled and chopped
1 medium tomato, chopped
½ yellow bell pepper, chopped
3 green onions, finely chopped
½ teaspoon sea salt
¼ teaspoon fresh ground pepper
½ teaspoon dry dill
or
½ teaspoon dry tarragon
or
1 tablespoon fresh cilantro, minced
½ cup plain low-fat yogurt

In a serving bowl, toss cucumber, tomato, yellow bell pepper, and green onions. In a separate bowl, mix salt, fresh ground pepper, dill, and yogurt. Combine the yogurt dressing with the cucumber salad. Cover and place in the refrigerator. Marinate for at least 3 hours for the flavors to develop. Serve with whole-wheat garlic bread.

Rudy's summer salad has very little fat but is very tasty. The rainbow of vegetables provides minerals and antioxidants that are very beneficial to the skin and retard skin aging.

CHAPTER 36

Spiritual Growth

Spirituality, as I understand it, is the depth that comes from the confidence that you know your own soul. Perhaps another way to define spirituality is being at peace with yourself. Wouldn't it be wonderful if we could increase spirituality simply by the way we ate? Albert Einstein felt this was not only possible but very important for personal as well as planetary evolution. So did Gandhi, who said, "I do feel that spiritual progress does demand at some stage that we should cease to kill our fellow creatures for the satisfaction of our bodily wants."

A spiritual person is someone whose priority is to taste the elixir of God in the early ambrosial hours of every morning and to keep that elevated state of grace with himself or herself throughout the busy hours of the day. This person is a pure one. To be pure and to be able to meditate deeply or concentrate well requires a lower-frequency diet. That means no meat, fish, chicken, or eggs. In my view, a pure person eats nothing that can swim, run, or fly away. Not eating meat develops in you a higher taste. You begin to use food to feed your spirit, not just your body and mind.

What do you think about spirituality and food? Take some time to meditate on what the relationship between food and spirituality means to you.

A DIET FOR SPIRITUAL GROWTH

I once asked the master of yoga nutritional therapy, Yogi Bhajan, for a diet for spiritual growth. The one he sent me follows. Although it was specifically prescribed for me, it has worked for others as well. The diet is low in calories and you will lose weight by following it. But, more to the point, in a very short time, perhaps as little as forty days, you will also come to realize your own divine essence.

If you choose to follow this diet, I suggest that you set aside a very special time of contemplation, relaxation, and meditation in which to begin. Perhaps you can take a vacation for two weeks and go to a secluded spot, or take the time off at home. You can also start off with a ten-day holiday, and then try and follow the program as well as you can when you return to work for another thirty days. It is best to follow the diet for a total of forty days.

I've heard folks say upon ending a retreat like this that "it's time to go back to reality." To me, the feeling you get from this diet for spiritual growth, especially when it is combined with the practice of kundalini yoga, meditation, and prayer, is true reality. The rest is just mundane.

Breakfast
whole wheat toast with honey or jelly and cinnamon
1 banana
1 tablespoon raisins blended with ¾ cup pure water to make a drink

Cinnamon is a blood purifier and a general energizer, and bananas are relaxing and calming to the nervous system. Raisins are powerful antioxidants and a source of minerals and energy.

Midmorning snack
1 cup carrot juice

Carrot juice is beneficial for the eyes, organs, and tissues and is a powerful antioxidant.

Lunch
Mung beans and rice recipe (see page 80)

Midafternoon snack
Jalapeno milk (see page 142)

Dinner
Lettuce Soup
    ½ head butter lettuce
    3 cups pure water
    1 teaspoon Braggs Liquid Aminos

1 teaspoon extra virgin olive oil
5 cashews
5 walnuts
5 pistachios
5 almonds

Optional:
½ small white onion

Boil the butter lettuce and onion (optional) in water until well cooked. Do not strain; just add Braggs Liquid Aminos and extra virgin olive oil. Serve with nuts on the side or in the soup. Lettuce soup has a relaxant effect while providing omega-3 oil and protein, and it helps sustain the immune system.

Evening snack
Turmeric yogurt (prepare a paste of turmeric by cooking it for 5 minutes in a little water, then add a teaspoon to 1 cup nonfat yogurt). Turmeric is a powerful anti-inflammatory.

SUPPLEMENTS AND SPECIFIC NUTRIENTS
Primary
Everyone should take a high-potency multiple vitamin and mineral supplement, as explained in the fifth principle (see page 120).

HERBS
Primary
Royal Vitality-Herbal Gems: 2 caps at night with lettuce soup (See Appendix E, Resources). Royal Vitality is a general lifelong tonic.

Digest Rite-Herbal Gems: 2 caps at night with lettuce soup (See Appendix E, Resources). Digest Rite is a general anti-inflammatory and helps the digestive system.

Stress and Anxiety

Stress is defined as that point when your ability to perform is exceeded by the demand placed upon you. The demand can be known or unknown, conscious or not. Anxiety is a symptom of stress and can also be an emotional disorder of its own.

Chronic, unbalanced stress is responsible for over 70 percent of all visits to the doctor's office. If you add chronic pain, this figure rises to over 80 percent. The fact that tranquilizers are among America's most commonly prescribed drugs also highlights the epidemic of stress in this country.

Stress kills. It either helps cause, or worsens, every conceivable illness from heart disease and stroke to memory loss, chronic infections, and probably cancer. Most people I see in consultation, in workshops, or at my presentations agree that it is next to impossible to decrease the demands made on them in today's fast-paced world. So what can they do—and, more important, what can *you* do to alleviate stress?

Meditation, of course, is a very powerful way to activate your body's natural healing force. So is following the yoga nutritional therapy program. Signals of peace, love, and healing sent by the food you eat can go a long way toward moving you back to a high level of personal performance.

DIET

If you are near your stress limit, begin eating a diet composed of 50 to 75 percent raw foods. Fresh fruits and vegetables supply valuable compounds, such as vitamin C, ellagic acid, and quercetin, that scavenge and neutralize dangerous free radicals. Fruits and vegetables send soft signals to your genes, which then send positive healing signals throughout your body.

Stay away from high-alarm processed foods, which put undue stress on your healing system. These foods include artificial sweeteners, soft drinks, fried foods, junk foods, pork, red meat, white flour products, and foods containing preservatives or heavy spices. Eliminate dairy products from your diet for three weeks, and then reintroduce them slowly. Limit caffeine, and avoid mood-altering drugs.

SUPPLEMENTS AND SPECIFIC NUTRIENTS

Primary

Everyone should take a high-potency multiple vitamin and mineral supplement, as explained in the fifth principle (see page 120). In addition, to heal the negative effects of stress, I recommend taking the following nutrients:

Vitamin C: 3,000 to 10,000 mg per day. Vitamin C is very important for adrenal gland function, which produces antistress hormones.

Phosphatidylserine: 100 to 300 mg per day blocks the effects of cortisol, a dangerous stress chemical.

Coenzyme Q10: 100 mg per day to increase energy.

DHEA: 25 to 100 mg per day, depending on age, sex, and current DHEA blood level. As with any other hormone, you should take DHEA only under a doctor's supervision. DHEA blunts the production of the stress hormone cortisol.

HERBS

Secondary

Kava kava: 100 mg three times per day activates the effect of a relaxing chemical in the brain called gamma-aminobutyric acid (GABA). In a report of fifty-two patients with symptoms of stress, more than 80 percent of those taking kava kava rated the effects very good or good. Consult with your doctor before taking kava kava because of emerging concerns about possible side effects on the liver. Also, don't mix it with any mind-altering substances such as alcohol, recreational drugs, or tranquilizers. Kava kava should be used as part of a holistic program that examines the underlying causes of your anxiety.

Valerian root: 450 mg three times per day. Valerian root appears to work in the same way as kava kava; it affects the GABA receptors in the brain. Valerian root should be used as a natural bridge to recover your balance after stress. If you need to take valerian root for more than three days, please discuss it with your doctor. Valerian root is not to be mixed with prescription drugs because it can augment their effects. Don't drive or operate heavy machinery while taking valerian root.

Lavender: If you want a very pleasant, mild anxiety reducer or sleep aid, add 5 to 10 drops of lavender oil to your bath water, or simply diffuse the essential oil in your bedroom or any room in your home or office. To diffuse, follow the instructions on your aromatherapy kit. But perhaps the easiest way to gain the relaxing effects of lavender is to rub lavender massage oil on your arms, legs, and body.

Lavender, primarily in the form of oil, has often been the subject of scientific inquiry. It has been found to reduce several physiological parameters of stress by stimulating serotonin and inducing a feeling of calm and happiness.

JUICE

The Stress Melter
Makes 1 serving

¼ head lettuce, preferably butter lettuce, outer leaves removed
1 carrot
1 tomato
1 celery stalk

Optional: ½ cup ice

Wash and dry the lettuce, carrot, tomato, and celery. Juice all together, and pour over ice, if desired. Fresh juices are best consumed within 2 to 3 hours of preparation and should be refrigerated. Lettuce is high in potassium, phosphorus, and vitamin A. It has a sedative effect because of its naturally occurring endorphins and will quickly help to melt your stress away. Carrot, tomato, and celery are rich in antioxidants that have calming properties for your system.

RECIPE

Paola's Eggplant Rolls
Makes 4–6 servings

2 medium eggplants, cut into ½-inch slices
pinch of sea salt
10 to 12 slices fresh mozzarella cheese, ⅛ inch thick, cut in half
10 to 12 slices tofurella cheese, or provolone, ⅛ inch thick,
    cut in half
¼ cup pesto sauce
toothpicks
2 teaspoons extra virgin olive oil

Preheat oven to 350°F. Sprinkle each of the eggplant slices with a pinch of salt on one side, and lay on a baking sheet. Bake for 10 minutes, turn over and cook for another 10 minutes. Remove from oven, and let cool.

Fill each eggplant slice with a piece of mozzarella, a piece of tofurella, and ½ teaspoon of pesto. Roll the slice and close it with a toothpick. Place all rolls in a baking dish, sprinkle with the olive oil, and bake for 15 minutes. Serve warm.

Eggplant is an excellent source of fiber, is an appetite stimulant, a mild laxative and diuretic, and a good food for people with diabetes. It helps reduce cholesterol and arteriosclerosis, improves the immune system, and is also used for health recovery. All of these can be the consequences of too much stress.

Thyroid

Thyroid hormone is responsible for optimum metabolism in the body. When the thyroid gland's secretions are too high, the condition is called hyperthyroidism. Symptoms of this condition are an increased metabolism, fast pulse, anxiety, weight loss, and insomnia. As many as 12 percent of Americans have mild hyperthyroidism, according to *Harrison's Textbook of Internal Medicine.*

When the thyroid gland's secretions are too low, the condition is called hypothyroidism. A person will notice dry and flaky skin, poor hair and nail growth, slow reflexes and mentation, and weight gain. Thyroid deficiency may be due to the underproduction of thyroid hormones or the reduction in the hormone secreted by the pituitary gland that stimulates the thyroid.

DIET
A yoga nutritional therapy diet with the addition of iodine-rich sea vegetables, such as dulse and kelp, will help tonify your thyroid gland. Also emphasize beans, spinach, and seeds in your diet.

SUPPLEMENTS AND SPECIFIC NUTRIENTS
Primary
Everyone should take a high-potency multiple vitamin and mineral supplement, as explained in the fifth principle (see page 120).

If you have hyperthyroidism, you must be under the care of an endocrinologist. Therapies include surgery and medication.

To help the thyroid release additional hormone in hypothyroidism, take these supplements:

Zinc: 15 to 30 mg per day to help regulate thyroid function.

Vitamin C: 1,000 to 3,000 mg per day to support the immune system.

Secondary

Alpha-lipoic acid: 250 to 500 mg per day for cellular energy production.

Tyrosine: 300 to 1,000 mg per day. Tyrosine is an amino acid used in thyroid hormone production.

If you are clinically hypothyroid, you need to take thyroid hormone. See anti-aging section, page 166.

HERBS

Secondary

While there are no specific herbs that directly support the thyroid gland, a Longevity Green Drink (see Appendix E, Resources) or other green powder containing dulse, kelp, and Japanese sea vegetables may be useful. Add ½ scoop to smoothies or to the juice recipe below.

JUICE

Thyroid Surprise
Makes 1 serving

2 large carrots
1 cup spinach
1 teaspoon kelp powder
1 teaspoon brewer's yeast

Wash and dry the carrots and spinach, then juice them. Stir in the kelp and brewer's yeast. Fresh juices are best consumed within 2 to 3 hours of preparation and should be refrigerated.

The vegetables in this recipe are an excellent source of antioxidants, and kelp is the greatest source of iodine, the mineral that helps regulate thyroid function.

RECIPE

Thyroid Booster Salad
Makes 6 to 8 servings

5 cups pure water
1 cup dried wakame

6 ounces soba noodles
4 tablespoons cider vinegar
3 tablespoons soy sauce
2 teaspoons honey
¼ tablespoon sesame oil
1 green onion, chopped
1 cucumber, peeled, seeded, and sliced
½ cup thinly sliced carrots
½ red bell pepper, sliced into strips

Bring water to a boil. Add wakame and soba noodles, and continue to boil for 10 to 12 minutes. Drain noodles and let cool. Cut the wakame into thin strips 2 to 3 inches long by ⅛ inch wide.

To make salad dressing, whisk together vinegar, soy sauce, honey, and sesame oil.

Toss wakame strips, chopped onion, and soba noodles together with the dressing in a large salad bowl. Let marinate for 30 minutes in refrigerator. Then add cucumber, carrots, and red bell pepper. Toss and serve.

Wakame, like other seaweed, provides the body with over fifty different minerals and trace elements. It is excellent in aiding digestion, healing mucus membranes and joints, and optimizing thyroid function.

CHAPTER 39

Weight Loss

Obesity grew by 60 percent in the American population between 1991 and 2000. Twenty-seven percent of us are now considered obese, and 61 percent now qualify as overweight. That puts obesity at epidemic proportions in America. According to recent reports, obesity may be contributing more to our rising health care and drug costs than smoking and alcohol abuse combined. In fact, a study published in *Health Affairs* in 2002 reported that obesity is more harmful to the health than smoking or drinking.

Researchers say that obesity increases the costs of physician care by 36 percent and of medications by a whopping 77 percent. Moreover, being obese ages you by twenty years, putting a significantly overweight forty-year-old in the same risk category as a sixty-year-old for cancer, heart disease, and diabetes.

According to the American Diabetes Association, as waistlines expand, so do cases of type II adult onset diabetes. The American Diabetes Association predicts that the growing girth of the American public foreshadows an even larger increase in the number of cases of type II diabetes in the near future. Obesity is also now linked to certain cancers. In addition to the connection between obesity and colon cancer, we now know that overweight may significantly increase the risk of cancer of the pancreas. Pancreatic cancer is very hard to treat and kills nearly 29,000 Americans each year.

THE YOGA NUTRITIONAL THERAPY APPROACH TO WEIGHT LOSS
Once, a student in India went to see his guru because he needed advice on losing weight. The teacher gave him two eggplants of different sizes and told him that he was to eat them only when the large one became as small

as the little one and the little one grew as big as the large one. Being an obedient disciple, the man waited for a month, only drinking water. He returned a month later and said, "Sir, nothing happened."

The teacher said, "Throw them away. If they didn't change by now, they must be totally useless." By that time, however, the man was at his perfect weight and in excellent health.

Now, I'm not suggesting that you go on a total water fast for a month, but if you need to lose weight, the formula is this: drink more, eat less, and exercise. In the end, this is the only way to keep your weight stabilized. Americans are fat because they eat far more calories than they expend in their daily activities. Eating fewer calories is life extending and health promoting. It sends a very positive message to your genes.

To lose weight, you must observe portion size, as I discussed in detail in the seventh principle (see page 128 and Appendix B, Portions). Two other weight loss tips are never to eat standing up and to eat only light, nutritious snacks, such as a small organic apple, if you're hungry between meals.

Also, avoid processed foods and junk foods, and be careful of low-fat and nonfat snacks that are high in refined carbohydrates. Eliminate the use of artificial sweeteners, which have never been proved to help anybody lose weight and are GMO. Finally, many people report that they lose weight by cutting down or eliminating bread. I agree, and I recommend not eating bread if you want to lose weight. Its very high carbohydrate content can lead to weight gain. If you absolutely need to eat bread, make it pumpernickel, nine-grain, or rice bread, and eat only one piece per day during your weight loss diet period.

I always like to have a person who wants to lose weight begin with a short detoxifying fast, as described in the first principle (see page 70). Then I recommend broccoli, beets and beet greens, and raw carrots, which are all low in calories but quite filling. A cup of basmati rice can be eaten with these vegetables. It provides a small amount of carbohydrates, which are essential for the brain, and causes the kidneys to excrete toxins from the body. A monodiet of basmati rice cooked with lemon and turmeric, served with steamed vegetables, will help you shed pounds and leave you healthy and glowing.

OVERWEIGHT OR FIT?

I am often asked the difference between an overweight person and a fit one. An overweight person eats mostly refined food and most likely also eats meat in large quantities. Over 40 percent of their calories come from fat. They have at least 2 teaspoons of sugar daily, which stimulates their appetite. The overweight person subsequently makes more visits each year to the doctor for allergies, arthritis, sleep disorders, depression, cancer, heart disease, diabetes, and high blood pressure.

By contrast, a fit person eats more fresh produce, less meat, and less sugar and enjoys whole grains in moderation. He or she reaps the benefits of greater self-esteem, fewer accidents, less heartburn, higher energy, increased vitality, and longer life.

SUPPLEMENTS AND SPECIFIC NUTRIENTS

Primary

Everyone should take a high-potency multiple vitamin and mineral supplement, as explained in the fifth principle (see page 120).

There are no specific nutrients to help you lose weight. However, chromium is considered important in glucose metabolism and is part of my basic vitamin/mineral formula. Depending on your age and lab values, you may consider hormone replacement therapy to reduce body fat, or cholesterol-lowering nutrients to aid in reducing high blood cholesterol and lipids, which are possible complications of overweight.

HERBS

Secondary

Although there are no weight loss herbs, the herbal preparation known as Royal Vitality-Herbal Gems (see Appendix E, Resources) contains amalki, bibhitaki, and haritaki, which help increase metabolism and elimination, thus helping you lose weight. Royal Vitality must be used in conjunction with exercise and the suggestions described in this chapter. Take 2 capsules three times per day. There are no side effects.

JUICE

Morning Starter
Makes 1 serving

juice of ½ lemon
1 cup warm water

Pour lemon juice in water, and drink through a straw over a half-hour period, the first thing in the morning. When taken according to these guidelines, this simple drink will help detoxify the liver, colon, and blood. It will suppress appetite and act as a healing food.

RECIPE

The Yogis' Weight Loss Monodiet
Makes 4 servings

4 or 5 zucchinis, unpeeled
4 celery stalks
1 cup parsley leaves
1 sprig of mint
coarsely ground black pepper, to taste
¼ cup nonfat cottage cheese per serving

Wash, dry, and take ends off zucchinis and celery. Wash and dry parsley and mint. Steam zucchinis and celery for 15 minutes or until soft, then puree in a Vita-Mix or blender with parsley, mint, and ground black pepper. Serve with nonfat cottage cheese.

Eat only this food for 40 days. Eat as much as you like, but no more than three times per day. Besides helping to lose weight, this diet is excellent for cleaning the intestines and clearing your skin.

You may also drink Yogi Tea with this monodiet (see page 138).

CHAPTER 40

Women's Health: Fibrocystic Breast Disease, Menopause, Osteoporosis, Premenstrual Syndrome (PMS), and Uterine Fibroids

Since the beginning of time, women have been recognized as having special qualities to heal, bring new life, educate children, and keep traditions. These qualities are all crucial for any culture. What we are not usually taught in the West, however, is that for a woman to be able to manifest such positive influence she has to be in physical, mental, emotional, and spiritual balance.

Fibrocystic breast disease, menopause, osteoporosis, premenstrual syndrome (PMS), and uterine fibroids are all associated with the alarm signals sent by our Western lifestyle, which is high in fatty foods, stress, smoking, caffeine, and alcohol. Food is a woman's best medicine to heal and regain balance from these afflictions.

Yoga nutritional therapy foods that are very beneficial to women include watermelon, bananas, raisins, citrus fruits, plums, peaches, papayas, and dates. Specific vegetables vital to women's health include beets and beet greens, eggplants, and all other green vegetables. Nuts and raw, edible, cold-pressed almond oil are also considered invaluable for women to maintain maximum health. Because of their specific phytonutrient makeup and alkalinizing effect, all these fruits and vegetables balance a woman's metabolism and energy.

According to the ancient masters of yoga nutritional therapy, every woman should eat a meal of steamed vegetables each day. Soy is also very beneficial for women because of its high content of phytoestrogens and isoflavones, which protect against heart disease and limit the symptoms of menopause. Present research is shedding some new light on the effects of soy on women's health, so please check with your nutritionally oriented doctor before using it to treat any symptoms you have.

A very special herb for women's health is black cohosh, which you will see recommended for female health concerns in the following pages. Nine clinical trials have supported the benefits of this herb. It is the most widely used herb for the alleviation of menopausal complaints. Although black cohosh has been studied, how it works is still unknown.

FIBROCYSTIC BREAST DISEASE

Fribrocystic breast disease is a common concern among women, especially since it may be initially thought to be cancer. Cysts may be hereditary and are probably aggravated by hormonal imbalance.

DIET

Reduce your fat intake to 20 percent or less, eliminate caffeine, and switch to hormone-free meats and dairy while you make the transition to a plant-based diet. Pears are a traditional yoga nutritional therapy food used to treat and prevent growths in the breast and elsewhere, so eat pears regularly and drink pear juice to prevent fibrocystic breast disease.

SUPPLEMENTS AND SPECIFIC NUTRIENTS

Primary

Everybody should take a high-potency multiple vitamin and mineral supplement, as explained in the fifth principle (see page 120). In addition, if you have fibrocystic breast disease, I recommend the following nutrients:

Essential fatty acids: 1,000 mg per day. Essential fatty acids help balance hormones that have been found responsible for fibrocystic breast disease.

Vitamin C: 1,000 mg three times per day to help boost the immune system.

Evening primrose oil: 1,500 mg per day to possibly help reduce the size of the lumps.

Secondary
Coenzyme Q10: 100 mg per day to help provide intracellular energy to
remove toxins from the body and boost the immune system.

HERBS

Primary
Turmeric: 100 to 200 mg per day to provide a natural anti-inflammatory
effect. It may also be used in food.
Ginger: 500 mg twice per day is a natural healer and anti-inflammatory.
Ginger may also be used in food.

MENOPAUSE

The cessation of estrogen secretion by the ovaries is usually associated with
several side effects. Many of them can be quite unpleasant. They include
depression, skin and vaginal dryness, lack of libido, hot flashes, cognitive
disturbance, osteoporosis, and heart disease. The treatment of menopause
is undergoing rapid positive change. However, the one treatment that has
stood the test of time is nutritional therapy, which has proved that what a
woman eats can make her symptoms either worse or more tolerable.

DIET

If you want to reduce your symptoms of menopause, you should reduce fat,
caffeine, and alcohol in your diet. Make sure you increase your consumption of bioflavonoids by eating plenty of fruits and vegetables. Also, increase your intake of vitamin E, found in most nuts and in wheat germ. The
phytoestrogens contained in soy products are also very therapeutic for the
symptoms of menopause because they have a hormonal balancing effect.

SUPPLEMENTS AND SPECIFIC NUTRIENTS

Primary
Everybody should take a high-potency multiple vitamin and mineral supplement, as explained in the fifth principle (see page 120). In addition, to
alleviate the symptoms of menopause, I recommend taking the following
nutrients:

Vitamin C: 1,000 to 3,000 mg per day, to help reduce hot flashes and
boost the immune system.

Evening primrose oil: 3,000 mg per day. Primrose oil alleviates menopausal symptoms such as hot flashes.

Secondary
Coenzyme Q10: 100 mg per day to help with detoxification, increase your energy level, support adrenal gland function, and boost your immune system.

HERBS

Primary
Black cohosh: 40 mg twice per day is very beneficial in the treatment of female hormone problems. *Note:* Do not use black cohosh during pregnancy.
Quercetin: 2 mg per day to help with hot flashes.

Secondary
Licorice: 10 drops taken in an extract or by chewing on the root. Licorice has mild estrogen-like effects. However, if you have high blood pressure, you should not consume it.
Dong quai: 3 to 5 mg per day. Dong quai is the most often prescribed herbal remedy in Oriental medicine because it helps balance hormonal levels. It is usually available in preparations containing other herbal extracts as well as from your Oriental medicine practitioner or at your local health food store.

A special note about hormone replacement therapy and menopause
Forty percent of postmenopausal women use hormone replacement therapy. Until recently, doctors and patients considered it to be a life-saving fountain of youth, but that has changed with the increasing awareness that Premarin, the most commonly used form of conventional hormone replacement therapy, actually comes from the urine of a pregnant horse. Recent studies on the effects of hormone replacement therapy have also given cause for caution.

Although the answers aren't all in yet, especially regarding the prevention of osteoporosis, what is clear is that hormone replacement therapy is an individualized choice rather than a one-size-fits-all treatment, as was previously thought. Studies conducted at the Stanford University School of Medicine between 1993 and 1998, and published in the February 6, 2002, edition of the *Journal of the American Medical Association,* showed that women without symptoms of menopause, such as hot flashes, actually have a negative lifestyle response to hormone replacement therapy with Premarin. The side effects include breast tenderness and abnormal bleeding. Women with hot flashes, however, had improvements in their emotional well-being, including energy, physical activity, mental health, and level of depression. It was also noted that hormone replacement therapy did not protect against the development of heart disease, as was previously thought.

If you have any symptoms of menopause, I suggest that you consider natural hormone replacement therapy, such as Bi-est or Tri-est.

Some physicians believe that Tri-est, a mixture of three natural estrogens, is more natural, while others prefer Bi-est, a mix of two naturally occurring estrogens, estrol and estradiol. In either case, hormone replacement therapy involves the art as well as the science of practicing medicine, and you will need to discuss it with your doctor. For more information on natural hormone replacement therapy, see page 168.

OSTEOPOROSIS

Osteoporosis (bone thinning and loss) is one of the most painful side effects of menopause. It can also be dangerous, because thin bones are predisposed to break easily. In addition to proper nutrition and supplementation, regular cardiovascular exercise and weight-bearing exercise are crucial to prevent and treat osteoporosis.

DIET

Recommended yoga nutritional therapy foods to help prevent osteoporosis are those rich in bone-protective vitamin K, such as green leafy vegetables and broccoli. I also suggest that you reduce your total intake of dietary protein. The best way to accomplish that is to substitute vegetable protein for animal protein. This will also reduce your intake of saturated fat.

SUPPLEMENTS AND SPECIFIC NUTRIENTS

Primary

Everybody should take a high-potency multiple vitamin and mineral supplement, as explained in the fifth principle (see page 120). In addition, to prevent osteoporosis, I recommend taking the following:

Calcium: 2,000 mg per day to protect from bone loss.

Magnesium: 1,000 mg per day to protect from bone loss.

Boron: 3 mg per day to enhance calcium absorption.

HERBS

Primary

Black cohosh: 40 mg two times per day to help reduce inflammation and build strong bones.

Secondary

Longevity Green Drink (see Appendix E, Resources) or other green powder: ½ scoop per day. Contains trace minerals and trace elements, which are vital for healthy bone formation.

PREMENSTRUAL SYNDROME

Premenstrual syndrome (PMS) affects many women one to two weeks before the menstrual cycle. The symptoms may include abdominal bloating, backache, irritability, and anxiety.

DIET

Sesame oil is important to help stimulate your energy level during PMS and the menstrual cycle. Take 1 tablespoon of cold-pressed, uncooked, sesame oil per day in salads or soups.

Ginger is particularly good for menstrual cramps and the general fatigue associated with PMS. Prepare it in tea (see page 141 for recipe), buy it ready-made (see Appendix E, Resources), or mix it with vegetables in a sauté. You may also eat it in a bowl of steamed vegetables.

Other foods that help alleviate PMS symptoms are mangoes, and onions, ginger, garlic, and turmeric cooked together in stir-fries or soups.

SUPPLEMENTS AND SPECIFIC NUTRIENTS

Primary

Everybody should take a high-potency multiple vitamin and mineral supplement, as explained in the fifth principle (see page 120). In addition, for PMS, I recommend taking the following:

Black currant oil: 1,000 mg per day.

or

Flaxseed oil: 1,000 mg per day, to help reduce inflammation.

HERBS

Primary

Black cohosh: 40 mg two times per day is very beneficial in the treatment of female hormonal problems. *Note:* Do not use black cohosh during pregnancy.

Secondary

Dong quai: 3 to 15 mg per day. Dong quai is the most often prescribed herbal remedy in Oriental medicine because it helps balance hormone levels. Dong quai is usually available in preparations containing other herbal extracts as well as from your Oriental medicine practitioner or at your local health food store.

Aloe vera: 1 to 2 ounces once or twice a day. May be taken as a juice in the treatment of PMS. It helps with irritability and cramps.

UTERINE FIBROIDS

Uterine fibroids are benign growths that form in the uterus. They are estimated to affect 20 to 30 percent of all women between their late thirties and early forties.

DIET

Although it has not yet been substantiated by scientific evidence, I suspect that one of the most likely causes of uterine fibroids is the elevated hormonal content of meats and dairy. Therefore, I recommend that you eat only hormone-free animal products as you make the transition to a plant-based diet, rich in organically grown fruits and vegetables, and soy foods. You should also limit your overall fat intake to no more than 20 percent.

Pears are a traditional yoga nutritional therapy food to treat and prevent benign growths, so eat pears regularly.

SUPPLEMENTS AND SPECIFIC NUTRIENTS

Primary

Everybody should take a high-potency multiple vitamin and mineral supplement, as explained in the fifth principle (see page 120). I know of no specific nutrients for uterine fibroids. However, the following are important for overall health:

Vitamin C: 3,000 mg per day. Vitamin C boosts the immune system and is a powerful antioxidant.

Secondary
Alpha-lipoic acid: 100 mg per day. Alpha-lipoic acid has a balancing effect on the cells lining the uterus.
Coenzyme Q10: 100 mg per day to boost the immune system.

HERBS

Primary
Black cohosh: 40 mg two times per day has proved useful to balance the female reproductive system. *Note:* Do not use black cohosh during pregnancy.

JUICE

Sweet Magnesium Bone-Strengthening Smoothie
Makes 1 serving

½ pint blackberries
1 ripe banana
1 tablespoon brewer's yeast
1 cup soy milk

Wash and dry the berries. Peel the banana, and blend with remaining ingredients until smooth. Drink within 2 to 3 hours of preparation. Also, be sure to refrigerate the smoothie if you do not drink it immediately.

RECIPE

White Turnip Fast for PMS and menopausal stress relief

Go on a five- to seven-day fast of white turnips and their greens, plus at least 8 glasses of water per day. Steam the white turnips and their greens. Peel turnips and mash them with the greens. Add a precooked mixture of turmeric, black pepper, and ½ tablespoon of edible raw almond oil. Mix well—it should have a pudding-like consistency. You can repeat this short fast once a month if desired.

Turnips, also known as underground apples, will rebalance a woman's glandular system. They contain high amounts of calcium and potassium, which reduce the negative effects associated with PMS and menopause.

The Phytonutrient Effects of Common Foods

Foods	Phytonutrient	Effect
Garlic	Allyl sulfides	Eliminate cancer, lower cholesterol
Carrots, orange vegetables	Carotenoids	Neutralize free radicals
Fruit	Ellagic acid	Destroy cancer
Fruit, plus tea	Flavonoids	Antioxidants
Soy foods	Isoflavones	Decrease cancer risk
Cruciferous vegetables	Isothiocynates (sulforaphane)	Protect DNA
Citrus fruits	Limonene	Excrete carcinogens

Portion Sizes of Foods by Categories
Courtesy of Luz-Elena Shearer, MS, RD, CDE

Portion sizes listed below have been standardized by the American Dietetic Association. Please remember that individual servings may vary according to your caloric needs. All portion sizes correspond to serving sizes, except for meat portions. For information regarding your specific meal plan I suggest you consult a Registered Dietitian.

All foods listed are ready to eat or measured after cooking.

BEANS, PEAS, AND LENTILS LIST (STARCH GROUP, WHICH INCLUDES GRAINS, BEANS, AND STARCHY VEGETABLES)

Each portion contains approximately 15 grams carbohydrate, 3 grams protein, 0–1 grams fat, which total about 80 calories.

(Beans, peas, and lentils count as 1 starch portion, plus 5–7 gm of protein like an oz. of very lean meat.)

Beans and peas (garbanzo, pinto, mung, kidney and white, split, black-eyed)	1/2 cup
Lima beans	2/3 cup
Lentils	1/2 cup
Miso *	3 Tbsp

*Contains 400 mg or more of sodium per portion

BREAD LIST (STARCH GROUP, WHICH INCLUDES GRAINS, BEANS, AND STARCHY VEGETABLES)

Each portion contains approximately 15 grams carbohydrate, 3 grams protein, 0–1 grams fat, which total about 80 calories.

Bagel	(1 oz)
Bread, reduced-calorie	2 slices (1 oz)
Bread, whole-wheat, pumpernickel, rye	1 slice (1 oz)
Bread sticks, crisp, 4 in. long x 1/2 in	2 (2/3 oz)
English muffin	1
Pita, 6 in. across	1
Raisin bread, unfrosted	1 slice (1 oz)
Roll, small (whole wheat)	1 (1 oz)
Tortilla, corn, 6 in. across	1
Tortilla, flour, 6 in. across	1
Waffle, 4 in. square, reduced-fat whole grain	1

CARBOHYDRATES OTHER THAN FRUIT, MILK, OR STARCH GROUPS

(SEE also the Fruit, Milk, and Starch Groups, which contain carbohydrate.)

Each portion contains approximately 15 grams carbohydrate

Honey	1 Tbsp	1 carbohydrate
Hummus	1/3 cup	1 carbohydrate, 1 fat
Yogurt, frozen, low-fat, fat-free	1/3 cup	1 carbohydrate, 0–1 fat
Yogurt, frozen, fat-free, no sugar added	1/2 cup	1 carbohydrate
Yogurt, low-fat with fruit	1/3 cup	1 carbohydrates, 0–1 fat

CEREALS/GRAINS LIST (STARCH GROUP, WHICH INCLUDES GRAINS, BEANS, AND STARCHY VEGETABLES)

Each portion contains approximately 15 grams carbohydrate, 3 grams protein, 0–1 grams fat, which total about 80 calories.

Bran cereals	1/2 cup
Bulgur	1/2 cup
Cereals, NATURAL	1/2 cup
Cereals, unsweetened, ready-to-eat	1/2 cup
Cornmeal (dry)	3 Tbsp
Couscous	1/3 cup
Flour (dry) whole	3 Tbsp
Granola, low-fat	1/4 cup
Grape-Nuts®	1/4 cup
Grits	1/2 cup
Kasha	1/2 cup
Millet	1/4 cup
Muesli	1/4 cup

Oats	1/2 cup
Pasta	1/2 cup
Puffed cereal	1 cup
Rice milk	1/2 cup
Rice, brown or Basmati	1/3 cup
Shredded Wheat ®	1/2 cup
Wheat germ	3 Tbsp

CRACKERS/SNACKS LIST (STARCH GROUP, WHICH INCLUDES GRAINS, BEANS, AND STARCHY VEGETABLES)

Each portion contains approximately 15 grams carbohydrate, 3 grams protein, 0–1 grams fat, which total about 80 calories.

Matzoh	3/4 oz
Popcorn (popped, no fat added or low-fat microwave)	3 cup
Pretzels	3/4 oz
Whole-wheat crackers, no fat added	2–5 (3/4 oz)

FATS LIST (FAT GROUP)

Each portion contains approximately 5 grams fat,
which total about 45 calories.

Fats are divided into three groups, based on the main type of fat they contain: monounsaturated, polyunsaturated, or saturated fat. Small amounts of monounsaturated and polyunsaturated fats in the foods we eat are linked with good health benefits. Saturated fats are linked with heart disease and cancer.

MONOUNSATURATED FAT LIST:

Avocado, medium	1/8 (1 oz)
Oil (canola, olive, peanut)	1 tsp
Olives: ripe (black)	8 large
green, stuffed *	10 large
Nuts	
Almonds, cashews	6 nuts
Mixed (50% peanuts)	6 nuts
Peanuts	10 nuts
Pecans	4 halves
Peanut butter, smooth or crunchy	2 tsp
Sesame seeds	1 Tbsp
Tahiti paste	2 tsp

POLYUNSATURATED FAT LIST:

Nuts, walnuts, English	4 halves
Salad dressing: regular *	1 Tbsp
Reduced-fat	2 Tbsp
Seeds: pumpkin, sunflower	1 Tbsp

SATURATED FAT LIST*

Butter: stick	1 tsp
whipped	2 tsp
reduced-fat	1 Tbsp
Chitterlings, boiled	2 Tbsp (1/2) oz
Coconut, shredded	2 Tbsp
Cream cheese: reduced-fat	2 Tbsp (1 oz)

* Saturated fats can raise blood cholesterol levels.

FRUIT LIST (FRUIT GROUP, INCLUDES FRESH, DRIED, AND FROZEN)

Each portion contains approximately15 grams of carbohydrate, which total about 60 calories.

Apple, unpeeled, small	1 (4 oz)
Applesauce, unsweetened	1/2 cup
Apples, dried	4 rings
Apricots, fresh	4 whole (5 oz)
Apricots, dried	8 halves
Banana, small	1 (4 oz)
Blackberries	3/4 cup
Blueberries	3/4 cup
Cantaloupe, small	1/3 melon (11 oz) or 1 cup cubes
Cherries, sweet, fresh	12 (3 oz)
Dates	3
Figs, fresh	1 large or 2 medium (3 oz)
Figs, dried	1
Fruit cocktail	1/2 cup
Grapefruit, large	1/2 (11 oz)
Grapes, small	17 (3 oz)
Honeydew melon	1 slice (10 oz) or 1 cup cubes
Kiwi	1 (3 1/2 oz)
Mango, small	1/2 fruit (5 oz) or 1/2 cup
Nectarine, small	1 (5 oz)

Orange, small	1 (6 oz)
Papaya	1/2 fruit (8 oz) or 1 cup cubes
Peach, medium, fresh	1 (6 oz)
Pear, large, fresh	1/2 (4 oz)
Pineapple, fresh	3/4 cup
Plums, small	2 (5 oz)
Prunes, dried	3
Raisins	2 Tbsp
Raspberries	1 cup
Strawberries	1 cup whole berries
Tangerines, small	2 (8 oz)
Watermelon	1 slice (13 oz) or 1 cup cubes

FRUIT JUICE LIST (FRUIT GROUP, THESE ARE ABSORBED FROM YOUR DIGESTIVE SYSTEM ALMOST IMMEDIATELY AFTER CONSUMPTION—VERY FAST AND CONCENTRATED ENERGY.)

Each portion contains approximately 15 grams of carbohydrate, which total about 60 calories.

Apple juice/cider	1/2 cup
Cranberry juice cocktail	1/3 cup
Cranberry juice cocktail, reduced-calorie	1 cup
Fruit juice blends, 100% juice	1/3 cup
Grape juice	1/3 cup
Grapefruit juice	1/2 cup
Orange juice	1/2 cup
Pineapple juice	1/2 cup
Prune juice	1/3 cup

GRAINS (SEE CEREALS/GRAINS LIST.)
LENTILS (SEE BEANS, PEAS, AND LENTIL LIST.)
MEAT/PROTEIN AND SUBSTITUTES LIST

Meats and Protein Substitutes are divided into four categories: Very lean, Lean, Medium-fat, and High-fat meats based on the amount of fat they contain. A meal planning tip is to bake, roast, broil, grill, poach, steam, or boil meats rather than frying them. Also, place meat on a rack so the fat will drain off during cooking.

VERY LEAN MEAT/PROTEIN SUBSTITUTE LIST

Each ounce or quantity indicated in the following list contains 0 grams carbohydrate, 7 grams protein, 0–1 grams fat, which total about 35 calories. *Note* that your portion size may be 3 to 4 oz, in which case you would multiply the protein and fat grams by the amount of your portion size. (Example: 3 oz fish portion has 21 gm of protein and 0–3 gm of fat.)

Poultry:
  Chicken or turkey (white meat, no skin), Cornish hen (no skin)   1 oz
Fish
  Fresh or frozen cod, flounder, haddock, halibut, trout; tuna fresh or canned in water   1 oz
Game:
  Duck or pheasant (no skin), venison, buffalo, Ostrich   1 oz
Cheese with 1 gram or less fat per ounce:
  Nonfat or low-fat cottage cheese   1/4 cup
  Fat-free cheese   1 oz
Other: Processed sandwich meats with 1 gram or less fat
  Per ounce, such as deli thin, shaved meats, chipped
  Beef *, turkey ham   1 oz
  Egg whites   2
  Egg substitutes, plain   1/4 cup
  Hot dogs with 1 gram or less fat per ounce   1 oz
  Kidney (high in cholesterol)   1 oz
  Sausage with 1 gram or less fat per ounce   1 oz

  Count as one very lean meat and one starch exchange

  Beans, peas, lentils (cooked)   1/2 cup
*= 400 mg or more sodium per exchange.

LEAN MEAT/PROTEIN SUBSTITUTE LIST
Each ounce or quantity indicated in the following list contains 0 grams carbohydrate, 7 grams protein, 3 grams fat, which total about 55 calories. *Note* that your portion size may be 3 to 4 oz, in which case you would multiply the protein and fat grams by the amount of your portion size. (Example: 3 oz fish portion has 21 gm of protein and 9 gm of fat.)

Beef:
  USDA Select or Choice grades of lean beef trimmed of fat, such as round, sirloin, and flank steak; tenderloin; roast (rib, chuck, rump); steak (T bone, porterhouse, cubed), ground round   1 oz
Pork:
  Lean pork, such as fresh ham; canned, cured, or boiled Ham; Canadian bacon *; tenderloin, center loin chop   1 oz

Lamb:
    Roast, chop, leg   1 oz
Veal:
    Lean chop, roast   1 oz
Poultry:
    Chicken, turkey (dark meat, no skin), chicken (white meat, with skin), do-
    mestic duck or goose (well-drained of fat, no skin)   1 oz
Fish:
    Herring (not creamed or smoked)   1 oz
    Oysters   6 medium
    Salmon (fresh or canned), catfish   1 oz
    Sardines (canned)   1 oz
Game:
    Goose (no skin), rabbit   1 oz
Cheese:
    4.5%-fat cottage cheese   1/4 cup
    Grated Parmesan   2 Tbsp
    Cheese with 3 grams or less fat per ounce   1 oz

MEDIUM-FAT MEAT/PROTEIN SUBSTITUTE LIST

Each ounce or quantity indicated in the following list contains 0 grams carbohydrate, 7 grams protein, 5 grams fat, which total about 75 calories. *Note* that
your portion size may be 3 to 4 oz, in which case you would multiply the protein and fat grams by the amount of your portion size. (Example: 3 oz fish portion has 21 gm of protein and 15 gm of fat.)

Beef:
    Most beef products fall into this category (ground beef, meatloaf, corned
    beef, short ribs, Prime grades or meat trimmed of fat, such as prime rib)
    1 oz
Pork
    Top loin, chop, Boston butt, cutlet   1 oz
Lamb:
    Rib roast, ground   1 oz
Veal:
    Cutlet (ground or cubed, unbreaded)   1 oz
Poultry:
    Chicken (dark meat, with skin), ground turkey or ground chicken, fried
    chicken (with skin)   1 oz
Fish:
    Any fried fish product   1 oz

Cheese: With 5 grams or less fat per ounce (1 slice)

Feta	1 oz
Mozzarella	1 oz
Ricotta	1/4 cup (2 oz)
Soy Cheese	1 oz

Other:

Egg (high in cholesterol, limit 3 per week)	1
Sausage with 5 grams or less fat per ounce	1 oz
Soy milk	1 oz
Tempeh	1/4 cup
Tofu	4 oz or 1/2 cup

HIGH-FAT MEAT/PROTEIN SUBSTITUTE LIST

Each ounce or quantity indicated in the following list contains 0 grams carbohydrate, 7 grams protein, 8 grams fat, which total about 100 calories. *Note* that your portion size may be 3 to 4 oz, in which case you would multiply the protein and fat grams by the amount of your portion size. (Example: 3 oz. fish portion has 21 gm of protein and 24 gm of fat.)

Remember these items are high in saturated fat, cholesterol, and calories and may raise blood cholesterol levels if eaten on a regular basis.

Cheese: All regular cheeses, such as American*, cheddar, Monterey Jack, Swiss   1 oz

- Count as one high-fat meat plus two fat exchanges.

Peanut butter (contains unsaturated fat)	2 Tbsp
Almond butter (contains unsaturated fat)	2 Tbsp
Cashew butter (contains unsaturated fat)	2 Tbsp

*= 400 mg or more sodium per exchange

MILK LIST (MILK/YOGURT GROUP)

SKIM/VERY LOW-FAT MILK

Each portion in the following list contains 12 grams carbohydrate, 8 grams protein, 0–3 grams fat, which total about 90 calories. *Note:* 1 cup is 8 oz.

Fat-free milk	1 cup
1/2 % milk	1 cup

1 % milk	1 cup
Fat-free or low-fat buttermilk	1 cup
Evaporated fat-free milk	1/2 cup
Fat-free dry milk	1/3 cup dry
Plain nonfat milk	1/3 cup dry
Nonfat or low-fat fruit-flavored yogurt sweetened with a nonnutritive sweetener	1 cup

REDUCED OR LOW-FAT MILK

Each portion in the following list contains 12 grams carbohydrate, 8 grams protein, 0–3 grams fat, which total about 90 calories. *Note*: 1 cup is 8 oz.

2 % milk	1 cup
Plain low-fat yogurt	3/4 cup
Sweet acidophilus milk	1 cup
Soy Milk (Varies in protein, carbohydrate and fat from cow's milk)	1 cup

PEAS (SEE BEANS, PEAS, AND LENTIL LIST.)
PROTEIN (SEE MEAT/PROTEIN LIST OR BEANS, PEAS, AND LENTIL LIST.)
STARCH (SEE BEANS, PEAS, AND LENTILS OR BREAD OR GRAINS OR STARCHY VEGETABLES LISTS.)
STARCHY VEGETABLES (SEE VEGETABLE LIST.)
VEGETABLE LIST (INCLUDES LOW CARBOHYDRATE AND HIGH CARBOHYDRATE STARCHY VEGETABLES)

LOW CARBOHYDRATE VEGETABLES

Vegetables that contain small amounts of carbohydrates and calories are on this list. *One vegetable portion is approximately 5 grams carbohydrate, 2 grams protein, 0 grams fat, which total at most 25 calories.* Vegetables contain important nutrients. In general, one vegetable exchange is:

- 1/2 cup of cooked vegetables or vegetable juice
- 1 cup or raw vegetables.

Artichoke
Artichoke hearts
Asparagus
Beans (green, wax, Italian)
Bean sprouts

Beets
Broccoli
Brussels sprouts
Cabbage
Carrots
Cauliflower
Celery
Cucumber
Eggplant
Green onions or scallions
Greens (collard, kale, mustard, turnip)
Kohlrabi
Leeks
Mixed vegetables (without corn, peas, or pasta)
Mushrooms
Okra
Onions
Pea pods
Peppers (all varieties)
Radishes
Salad greens (endive, escarole, lettuce, romaine, spinach)
Sauerkraut *
Spinach
Summer squash
Tomato
Tomatoes, canned
Tomato sauce *
Tomato/vegetable juice *
Turnips
Water chestnuts
Watercress
Zucchini

*= 400 mg or more sodium per exchange

STARCHY VEGETABLES

Each portion contains approximately 15 grams carbohydrate, 3 grams protein, 0–1 grams fat, which total about 80 calories.

(Beans, peas and lentils count as 1 starch portion, plus 5–7 gm of protein like an oz of very lean meat.)

Baked beans	1/3 cup
Corn	1/2 cup
Corn on cob, medium	1 (5 oz)
Mixed vegetables with corn, peas, or pasta	1 cup
Peas, green	1/2 cup
Plantain	1/2 cup
Potato, baked or boiled	1 small (3 oz)
Potato, mashed	1/2 cup
Squash, winter (acorn, butternut, pumpkin)	1 cup
Yam, sweet potato, plain	1/2 cup

Samples of Vegetarian Sources of Protein and Other Products, Listed by Manufacturer

BOCA

Boca burgers

Boca burgers are meatless, non-GMO soy protein burgers that contain 75 percent less fat than a ground beef hamburger.

One burger contains

16 grams protein (130 calories)
11 grams carbohydrate
2.5 grams total fat, of which 1 gram is saturated; less than 5 grams cholesterol

By contrast, cooked ground beef contains 13 grams fat, 210 calories, and 70 mg cholesterol per serving. Boca burger has six different varieties of veggie burger, including my favorite, the salsa burger.

For more information, log on to www.bocaburger.com

GALAXY FOODS

Soycheese

A natural alternative to cheese made with organic tofu. It comes in many different flavors, including mozzarella.

One slice contains

4 grams protein (40 calories)
1 gram carbohydrate
2 grams fat, with 0 saturated and 0 cholesterol

For more information, log on to www.galaxyfoods.com

LIGHTLIFE

Smart deli bologna

Three slices contain

10 grams protein (50 calories)
2 grams carbohydrate
0 gram fat

Lightlife also makes other vegetarian deli slices, such as ham and turkey. They also offer cholesterol-free hot dogs with 9 grams of protein per serving. Lightlife has been committed to making vegetarian foods since 1979. They contribute five percent of their profits to organizations that work to protect children, human rights, the environment, economic justice, and world peace. If you want to learn more about them, their Web site is www.lightlife.com

MORI-NU

Mori-Nu tofu (organic and non-GMO)

A 3-oz serving contains

6 grams protein (35 calories)
1 gram carbohydrate
0.5 gram fat

As you are aware, tofu contains a full spectrum of naturally occurring soy isoflavones, including genistein. It is an excellent food for heart health and cancer prevention. To learn more about Mori-Nu, which I consider a very responsible company, log on to www.morinu.com to find tofu tips, recipes, and additional product information.

VEGGIE PATCH

Veggie patch veggitinos

This is a vegetarian meatball substitute that is ideal for pasta or to eat with tomato sauce and vegetables. In addition to being a good protein source, this product contains probiotics, a source of special fibers, which can significantly promote natural balance of the digestive system. Desirable bacteria use these fibers as an energy source, stimulating their metabolism and increasing their activity, leading to a healthier digestive tract. At the same time, the presence of less desirable bacteria is significantly reduced.

5 "meatballs" contain

15 grams protein (120 calories)
13 grams carbohydrate

2.5 grams total fat, with 0 cholesterol and 0 saturated fat

Visit Veggie Patch at www.veggiepatch.com

WHITE WAVE

Tempeh is a non-GMO organic product that contains soy, barley, millet, and brown rice. There is a wide assortment of tempeh products, including five-grain, sea vegetable, and soy rice.

White Wave soymilk (organic and non-GMO)

One cup contains

7 grams protein (100 calories)
8 grams carbohydrate
4 grams fat

White Wave tempeh (organic and non-GMO)

Contains

12 grams protein (140 calories)
4 grams total fat
15 grams carbohydrate

White Wave baked tofu (organic and Non-GMO)

White Wave has seven different styles of baked tofu, ranging from garlic herb Italian to teriyaki Oriental. The nutrient content varies:

8–13 grams protein (75–120 calories)
3–6 grams carbohydrate
3–8 grams fat

These delicious products serve as a major staple of my diet. Our nutritionist recommends them highly to my patients.

White Wave has several other products as well. Log on to their Web site www.silkissoy.com to learn more.

YOGI TEA

For the last 20 years, Yogi Tea has developed therapeutic teas based on the ancient principles of yoga and yoga nutritional therapy. Their teas are available at most health food stores or online at www.yogitea.com

Samples of their teas include Breathe Deep Tea, Echinacea Special Formula Tea, Woman's Formula Tea, Ginger Tea, Green Tea with Kombucha, and many others.

YVES

Yves veggie burger (organic and non-GMO)

Contains

16 grams protein (120 calories)
2 grams total fat
9 grams carbohydrate

This is also an excellent source of high-quality protein made with non-GMO soy. It is preservative free and costs less than $1.00 per burger.

Yves deli slices (organic and non-GMO)

Four slices contains

13 grams protein (80 calories)
1 gram total fat
4 grams carbohydrate

This tasty product is avery good source of protein and is great for a snack.

Yves breakfast links (organic and non-GMO)

Two links contains

11 grams protein (70 calories)
2 grams total fat
3 grams carbohydrate

Yves also makes non-GMO, preservative-free, cholesterol-free, high-protein veggie turkey, ham, salami, bologna, pizza pepperoni, and Canadian veggie bacon. You can check their Web site by logging on to www.yvesveggie.com.

APPENDIX D

Equipment and Utensils

To make the transition to a food-as-medicine lifestyle requires a few simple gadgets. Beyond the basic pots and pans, you'll want to have a blender, a food processor, and a rice cooker.

At times I've mentioned a Vita-Mix (*www.vitamix.com*), which can serve as a blender and a food processor in one. A Vita-Mix machine has a motor almost as powerful as a good lawn mower, so you know it can handle anything in the kitchen, including making almond butter from scratch. It also can make soups, juices, and natural ice cream. If you visit any of the many natural juice stores springing up around the country, you will notice they use a Vita-Mix. You are going to need a blender and food processor anyway, and this machine serves both those functions.

A rice cooker comes in two home-use sizes, large and small, depending on the size of your family. When I was single, I had a 1-liter rice cooker that made six servings of rice or another grain. When Kirti and I married, we got a larger one. The larger of the two holds almost 2 liters of water and makes ten servings. Make sure you get a rice cooker with a vegetable container/strainer that fits over the liquid. In this way you can cook rice and steam vegetables at the same time, or do either process alone.

Resources

CLEAN PROTEIN

Coleman Natural Products Inc.
5140 Race Court
Denver, CO 80216
Phone: (303) 297-9393
Web site: coleman@colemannatural.com

DHARMA SINGH KHALSA, M.D.

To schedule a consultation with Dharma Singh Khalsa, M.D., or to learn more about his work and speaking schedule, please contact:

Dharma Singh Khalsa, M.D.
2420 N. Pantano Road
Tucson, AZ 85715
Phone: (520) 749-8374
Fax: (520) 296-6640
e-mail: info@drdharma.com
Web site: www.drdharma.com

or

The Alzheimer's Prevention Foundation
2420 N. Pantano Road
Tucson, AZ 85715
Phone: (520) 749-8374
Fax: (520) 296-6640
e-mail: info@alzheimersprevention.org
Web site: www.alzheimersprevention.org

GOVERNMENT

To have a positive influence on the future of the planet, tell these organizations how you feel and what you want to see happen.

U.S. Department of Agriculture
Web site: www.usda.gov/biotechnology

U.S. Environmental Protection Agency
Web site: www.epa.gov/pesticides/biopesticides

U.S. Food and Drug Administration
Web site: www.fda.gov/oc/biotech/default.htm

U.S. House of Representatives
Web site: www.house.gov

U.S. Senate
Web site: www.senate.gov

The President of the United States
Web site: www.whitehouse.gov

MAGAZINES

Aquarian Times
Web site: www.aquariantimesmagazine.com

Natural Health
Web site: www.naturalhealth.com

New Age Journal
Web site: www.newage.com

Total Health Magazine
Web site: www.totalhealthmagazine.com

Vegetarian Times
Web site: www.vegetariantimes.com

Yoga Journal
Web site: www.yogajournal.com

NATIONAL ORGANIC GROCERY STORES

Trader Joe's*
Web site: www.traderjoes.com

*About 50 percent organic

Wild Oats
A large selection of organic foods.
Web site: www.wildoats.com

Whole Foods Market
A large selection of organic foods.
Web site: www.wholefoods.com

NUTRITIONAL SUPPLEMENTS

To obtain Dr. Khalsa's line of nutritional supplements, including the Longevity
Green Drink, please contact
Web site: www.drdharma.com

To obtain the other supplements mentioned in this book, please contact
Vitamin Research Products
3579 Highway 50 East
Carson City, NV 89701
Phone: 1 (888) 234-0459
Web site: www.vrp.com

To Obtain Herbal Gems, please contact
www.yogitea.com

Optimum Health International, LLC
Specializing in pharmaceutical-grade nutriceuticals, vitamins, and
minerals.
257 E. Center Street
Manchester, CT 06040
1 (800) 228-1507
www.optimumhealth.com

ORGANIZATIONS
National
The following appear to be excellent sources of information and good
work. If you are interested in these topics, by all means contact the groups of
your choice. One small step to save the earth goes a long way.

Campaign to Label Genetically Engineered Foods
P.O. Box 55699
Seattle, WA 98155
Phone: (425) 771-4049
Web site: www.thecampaign.org

Center for Food Safety
66 Pennsylvania Ave, SE, Suite 302
Washington, DC 20003
Phone: (202) 547-9359
Web site: www.centerforfoodsafety.org

Center for Science in the Public Interest (CSPI)
1875 Connecticut Ave, NW, Suite 300
Washington, DC 20009
Phone: (202) 332-9110
Web site: www.cspinet.org

Citizens for Health
P.O. Box 2260
Boulder, CO 80306
Phone: 1 (800) 357-2211
Web site: www.citizens.org

Community Alliance with Family Farmers
P.O. Box 363
Davis, CA 95617
Phone: (916) 756-8518
Web site: www.caff.org

The Edmonds Institute
20319 92nd Ave West
Edmonds, WA 98020
Phone: (425) 775-5383
Web site: www.edmonds-institute.org

Environmental Working Group
1718 Connecticut Ave, NW, Suite 600
Washington, DC 20009
Phone: (202) 667-6982
Web site: www.ewg.org

Farm Animal Reform Movement (FARM)
P.O. Box 30654
Bethesda, MD 20824
Phone: 1 (888) farm-usa
Web site: www.farmusa.org

Food and Water
389 Rt 215

Walden, VT 05873
Phone: 1 (800) eat-safe
Web site: www.foodandwater.org

Friends of the Earth
1025 Vermont Ave, NW
Washington, DC 20005-6303
Phone: (202) 783-7400, (877) 843-8687
Fax: (202) 783-0444
Web site: www.foe.org

Foundation on Economic Trends
1660 L Street, NW, Suite 216
Washington, DC 20036
Phone: (202) 466-2823
Web site: www.biotechcentury.org

Greenpeace USA
564 Mission Street
P.O. Box 416
San Francisco, CA 94105
Phone: 1 (800) 326-0959
Web site: www.greenpeaceusa.org/ge/

This is the organization I'm most familiar with and support. They have a great website concerning the dangers of GMO foods: www.realfoodnow.org

Humane Society of the United States
2100 L Street, NW
Washington, DC 20037
Web site: www.hsus.org

The Life Extension Foundation
P.O. Box 229120
Hollywood, FL 33022
Phone: 1 (800) 544-4440
Web site: www.lef.org

The Life Extension Foundation publishes an outstanding journal for the general public and the professional. They also offer excellent supplements at a reasonable price.

Mothers and Others for a Livable Planet
40 West 20th Street

New York, NY 10011-4211
Phone: (212) 242-0010
Web site: www.igc.apc.org/mothers

Organic Consumers Association
6114 Highway 61
Little Marais, MN 55614
Phone: (218) 726-1443
Web site: www.purefood.org

Organic Farming Research Foundation
P.O. Box 440
Santa Cruz, CA 95061
Phone: (831) 426-6606
Website: www.ofrf.org

Vegetarian Source Online
Web site: www.VegSource.com

Physicians Committed for Responsible Medicine
5100 Wisconsin Ave, NW, Suite 404
Washington, DC 20016
Phone: (202) 686-2210
Web site: www.pcrm.org

Public Citizen Stop Food Irradiation Project
215 Pennsylvania Ave, SE
Washington, DC 20003
Web site: www.citizen.org/cmep

Union of Concerned Scientists
2 Brattle Square
Cambridge, MA 02238-5552
Phone: (617) 547-5552
Web site: www.ucsusa.org

International
Physicians and Scientists for Responsible Application of Science and
Technology (PSRAST)
Web site: www.pcrm.org

PESTICIDES

National Coalition Against the Misuse of Pesticides
701 E Street, SE, Suite 200
Washington, DC 20003
Phone: (202) 543-5450
Web site: www.ncamp.org

Pesticide Action Network of North America
49 Powell St, Suite 500
San Francisco, CA 94102
Phone: (415) 981-1771

SPAS FOR FASTING AND DETOXIFICATION

The Cleanse
P.O. Box 1515
Santa Cruz, NM
Phone: 1 (800) 563-3327
Web site: www.thecleanse.com

We Care Holistic Health Center
18000 Long Canyon Road
Desert Hot Spring, CA 92241
Phone: 1 (800) 888-2523
Web site: www.wecarespa.com

YOGA NUTRITIONAL THERAPY

To find a specialist in yoga nutritional therapy in your area, please contact:

International Kundalini Yoga Teachers Association
Box 4, Shady Lane
Espanola, NM 87532
Phone: (505) 753-0423
e-mail: ikyta@3ho.org
Web site: www.kundaliniyoga.com

Notes and References

PART ONE
The Cutting Edge of Medicine

Chapter 1: Spiritual Nutrition

Much of my inspiration for this chapter and this book came from the Food as Medicine conference sponsored by the Center for Mind/Body Medicine in Washington, DC. James Gordon, M.D., is the President.

Information about the transition into the Age of Aquarius is from the teachings of Yogi Bhajan. You can also read more about it in my book *Meditation as Medicine,* published by Fireside Books in 2002.

David Eisenberg's work, originally published in the *New England Journal of Medicine* in 1991, covers the surge in patients visiting alternative medicine practitioners. Recent articles about his work include the following:

Eisenberg DM, Kaptchuk TJ, Laine C, Davidoff F. Complementary and alternative medicine: an Annals series. *Ann Intern Med* 2001; 135:208.

Neal R. Report by David M. Eisenberg, M.D. On educational issues pertaining to complementary and alternative medicine in the United States. *J Altern Complement Med* 2001; 7 (Suppl 1):S41–3.

Neal R. Report by David M. Eisenberg, M.D. On complementary and alternative medicine in the United States: overview and patterns of use. *J Altern Complement Med* 2001; 7 (Suppl 1):S19–21.

Dr. Andrew Weil's seven basic principles of diet and health are discussed in his book *Eating Well for Optimum Health.* New York: Alfred Knopf, 2000.

Chapter 2: What Signals Are You Sending to Your Body?

Much of my research on how nutrition affects genetics, cell communication, and inflammation came from the outstanding documentation of the Life Extension Foundation. The published work and presentations I've heard by Jeffrey Bland, Ph.D., and David Heber, M.D., Ph.D., were also very useful. The following articles and books are good starting points for a serious student of this topic.

Review article

Life Extension Foundation. Chronic inflammation: the epidemic disease of aging. *Life Extension,* January 2002. www.lef.org/magazine

Monograph

Bland, Jeffrey. *Improving Intercellular Communication in Managing Chronic Illness.* Gig Harbor, Wash.: 1999. Functional Medicine Seminar Series Health Comm International, Inc. 1999.

Selected medical articles

Bland J. New functional medicine paradigm: health problems associated with dysfunctional intercellular communications. *Int J Integ Med* 1999;1:11–6.

Hubinette A, Cnattingius S, Ekbom A, de Faire U, Kramer M, Lichtenstein P. Birth weight, early environment, and genetics: a study of twins discordant for acute myocardial infarction. *Lancet* 2001,357(9273):1997–2001.

Ioannides C. Effect of diet and nutrition on the expression of cytochromes P450. *Xenobiotica* 1999;29:109–54.

Jacob R. Folate, DNA methylation, and gene expression: factors of nature and nurture. *Am J Clin Nutr* 2000;72:903–4.

Lee CK, Klopp RG, Weindruch R. Gene expression profile of aging and its retardation by calorie restriction. *Science* 1999;285:1390–3.

Lichtenstein P. Environmental and heritable factors in the causation of cancer. *N Engl J Med* 2000;343:78–85.

Sadee W. The human genome project pharmacogenomics. *Br Med J* 1999;319:1286.

Svedberg P, Lichtenstein P, Pedersen NL. Age and sex differences in genetic and environmental factors for self-rated health: a twin study. *J Gerontol B Psychol Sci Soc Sci* 2001;56:S171–8.

Terry P, Baron JA, Weiderpass E, Yuen J, Lichtenstein P, Nyren O. Lifestyle and endometrial cancer risk: a cohort study from the Swedish Twin Registry. *Int J Cancer* 1999;82:38–42.

Van Ommen G, Bakker E, Den Dunnen J. The human genome project and the future of diagnostics, treatment, and prevention. *Lancet* 1999;354:5–10.

Weindruch R. Caloric restriction and aging. *Sci Am* 1996;274:46–52.

Books

Bland, Jeffrey. *Genetic Nutritioneering.* Los Angeles: Keats Publishing, 1999.

Heber, David. *What Color Is Your Diet?* New York: Regan Books, HarperCollins, 2001.

Steingraber, S. *Living Downstream: An Ecologist Looks at Cancer and the Environment.* Reading, Mass.: Addison-Wesley, 1997.

Walford, Roy, and Lisa Walford. *The Anti-Aging Plan: Strategies and Recipes for Extending Your Healthy Years.* New York: Four Walls Eight Windows, 1994.

Web site to learn more about caloric restriction
www.infinitefaculty.org.sci.cr

Chapter 3: Phytonutrients: How Vegetables and Fruits Act As Medicine

The basic information presented in this chapter was gleaned from attending the annual educational program of the American Institute of Cancer Research (AICR) as well as reading the institute's extensive literature, much of it medically oriented. The AICR is the nation's third largest cancer charity and focuses exclusively on the link between diet and cancer. It provides a wide range of consumer education programs that have helped millions of Americans learn to make changes to reduce their risk of cancer. AICR also supports innovative research in cancer prevention and treatment at universities, hospitals, and research centers across the United States. The institute has provided over $57 million in funding for research in diet, nutrition, and cancer.

To learn more about The American Institute of Cancer research:

AICR
1759 R Street, NW
Washington, DC 20009
Web site: www.aicr.org
E-mail: pr@aicr.org
Medical articles
The Journal of Nutrition, Volume 131, No. 115, November 2001, is devoted exclusively to the topic of phytonutrient research. It can be found online at the following website: www.nutrition.org

Chapter 4: Vegetables as Medicine

General sources
The Life Extension Foundation publishes an excellent monthly magazine that highlights breaking news on new medical advances, including topics such as vegetables and fruit as medicine. Contact the foundation at 1-800-544-4440 or online at www.lef.org

General references

New diet-cancer research shows variety to be key to cancer prevention. AICR news release, July 17, 2001.

New evidence reveals how common foods can specifically target, strengthen the body's first line of defense against cancer. AICR news release, July 17, 2001.

Medical References

Talalay P, Fahey JW. Phytochemicals from cruciferous plants protect against cancer by modulating carcinogen metabolism. *J Nutr* 2001; 131:3027S–33S.

Gerber M. The comprehensive approach to diet: a critical review. *J Nutr* 2001;131:3051S–5S.

Brenner DE. Multiagent chemopreventive combinations. *J Cell Biochem* 2000; (Suppl)34:121–4.

Heber D, Bowerman S. Applying science to changing dietary patterns. *J Nutr* 2001;131:3078S–81S.

Vay Liang G, Wong D, Butrum R. *Diet, nutrition and cancer prevention.* *J Nutr* 2001;131:3121S–6S.

Block G. Fruit, vegetables, and cancer prevention: a review of the epidemiological evidence. *Nutr; Cancer* 1992;18:1–29.

General books

Yeager, Selene, and the Editors of *Prevention* Magazine. *The New Foods For Healing.* New York: Bantam Books, 1999.

Carper, Jean. *Food, Your Miracle Medicine.* New York: HarperCollins, 1993.

Chapter 5: Fruit as Medicine

Further information on fruit as medicine can be found in the publications of the Life Extension Foundation, as noted above. The information on food as yoga nutritional therapy (YNT) comes from the teachings of Yogi Bhajan:

Bhajan, Yogi. *The Ancient Art of Self-Healing.* Eugene, Ore.: West Anandpur Publishers, 1982.

General books

Yeager, Selene, and the Editors of *Prevention* Magazine. *The New Foods for Healing.* New York: Bantam Books, 1999.

Heber, David. *What Color Is Your Diet?* New York: Regan Books, Harper-Collins, 2001.

Medical articles

Barch DH, Rundhaugen LM, Stoner GD, Pillay NS, Rosche WA. Structure-function relationships of the dietary anticarcinogen ellagic acid. *Carcinogenesis* 1996;17:265–9.

Narayanan BA, Geoffroy O, Willingham MC, Re GG, Nixon DW. p53/p21(WAFI/CIPI) expression and its possible role in GI arrest and apoptosis in ellagic acid treated cancer cells. *Cancer Lett* 1999;136:215–21.

Bickford PC, Gould T, Briederick L, Chadman K, Pollock A, Young D, Shukitt-Hale B, Joseph J. Antioxidant-rich diets improve cerebellar physiology and motor learning in aged rats. *Brain Res* 2000;866:211–7.

Bickford PC, Shukitt-Hale B, Joseph J. Effects of aging on cerebellar noradrenergic function and motor learning: nutritional interventions. *Mech Ageing Dev* 1999;111:141–54.

Kontiokari T, Sundqvist K, Nuutinen M, Pokka T, Koskela M, Uhari M. Randomised trial of cranberry-lingonberry juice and lactobacillus GG drink for the prevention of urinary tract infections in women. *Br Med J* 2001;322:1571.

Knekt P, Jarvinen R, Reunanen A, Maatela J. Flavonoid intake and coronary mortality in Finland: a cohort study. *Br Med J* 1996;312:478–81.

Hertog MG, Feskens EJ, Hollman PC, Katan MB, Kromhout D. Dietary antioxidant flavonoids and risk of coronary heart disease: the Zutphen Elderly Study. *Lancet* 1993;342:1007–11.

Chapter 6: Beyond the Rainbow of Vegetables and Fruit

The research material for this chapter came from a variety of sources. My years of study with giants in the field of nutritional healing, such as Paavo Airola, Ph.D., Bernard Jenson, Ph.D., and Yogi Bhajan, Ph.D., have allowed me to obtain firsthand information on this subject. Beyond that, the following books and monographs have been very useful:

Superfoods: Sea vegetables, Micro algaes, Bee foods and more. Published by Wild Oats Markets, Boulder, Colo. 1996.

Wigmore, Ann. *The Sprouting Book.* 1986.

Wigmore, Ann. *The Wheat Grass Book.* 1985.

Carper, Jean. *Food, Your Miracle Medicine.* New York: HarperCollins, 1995.

Balch, James and Phyllis Balch. *Prescription for Natural Healing.* 1990.

Hunter, Beatrice Trum. *Grain Power.* New Canaan, Ct.: Keats Publishing, 1994.

Airola, Paavo. *How to Get Well.* Phoenix, Ariz.: Health Plus Publishers, 1974.

Cousins, Gabriel. *Conscious Eating.* Santa Rosa, Calif.: Vision Books International, 1994.

Sears, Barry. *The Soy Zone.* New York: Regan Books/HarperCollins, 2000.

Kushi, Michio. *One Peaceful World: Michio Kushi's Approach to Creating a Healthy and Harmonious Mind, Home, and World Community.* New York: St. Martin's Press, 1987.

Medical articles

Kushi L, Cunningham JE. The macrobiotic diet in cancer. *J Nutr* 131: 3056S–64S. (For the serious student, this review article has 98 references.)

Jacobs DR, Marquart L, Kushi LH. Whole grain intake and cancer: an expanded meta-analysis. *Nutr Cancer* 1998;30:85–96.

Jacobs DR, Meyer KA, Kushi LH. Is whole grain intake associated with reduced total and cause specific death rates in older women? The Iowa Women's Health Study. *Am J Public Health* 1999;89:322–9.

Slavin JL. Mechanisms on whole grain foods on cancer risks. *J Am Coll Nutr* 2000;19:300S–7S.

Teas J, Harbison ML, Gelman RS. Dietary seaweed and mammary carcinogenesis in rats. *Cancer Res* 1984;44:2758–61.

Nishino H. Cancer prevention by carotenoids. *Mutat Res* 1998;402:159–63.

Wassel F. Pharmacological ramifications of wheat. *Int J Integ Med* 2001; 3:6–11.

McKenna D. Green tea. *Choices Health Med* 2002;2:16–7.

McKay DL, Blumberg J. The role of tea in human health: an update. *J Am Col Nutr* 2002;21:1–13.

Chapter 7: From Pyramids to Principles

The concept of moving beyond pyramids to embrace principles of yoga nutritional therapy is an original idea of mine based on my years of study with my teacher, Yogi Bhajan. There are, however, several books and medical articles that highlight the nutritional benefits, or lack thereof, of each of the three main pyramids.

Monograph

Moving Towards a Plant Based Diet. Washington, D.C.: American Institute for Cancer Research, 2000. www.aicr.org

General books

Heber, David. *What Color Is Your Diet.* New York: Regan Books/HarperCollins, 2001.

Roizen, Michael, and John La Palma. *The Real Age Diet.* New York: HarperCollins, 2001.

Willett, Walter. *Eat, Drink, and Be Healthy.* New York: Simon and Schuster, 2001.

Medical articles

Simopoulos AP. The Mediterranean diets: what is so special about the diet of Greece? The scientific evidence. *J Nutr* 2001;131:3065S–73S.

Simopoulos AP. Omega-3 fatty acids in health and disease and in growth and development. *Am J Clin Nutr* 1991;54:438–63.

Joseph JA. Reversals of age-related declines in neuronal signal transduction, cognitive, and motor behavioral deficits with blueberries, spinach, or strawberry dietary supplementation. *J Neurosci* 1999;19:8114–21.

Mazur WM. Isoflavonoids and lignanes in legumes: nutritional and health aspects in humans. *J Nutr Biochem* 1998;9:193–200.

Weisburger JH. Mechanisms of action in antioxidants as exemplified in vegetables, tomatoes and tea. *Food Chem Toxicol* 1999;37:943–8.

Jang M, Cai I. Cancer chemopreventive activity of resveratrol, a natural product derived from grapes. *Science* 1997;275:218–20.

Chapter 8: The First Principle: Detoxify Your Body with Colon Therapy and Fasting

Most of the information for this chapter came from my own experience. I have experienced this type of program many times and have also interviewed many people who have done the same. The following books, however, may prove interesting.

Internal Cleansing. Monograph produced and published by Wild Oats Markets with headquarters in Boulder, Colo.; online at www.wildoats.com

Airola, Paavo. *How to Keep Slim and Young with Juice Fasting.* Phoenix, Ariz.: Health Plus Publishers, 1978.

Jensen, Bernard. *Tissue Cleansing Through Bowel Management.* Escondido, Calif.: Jensen Publishers, 1981.

Airola, Paavo. *Juice Fasting.* Phoenix, Ariz.: Health Plus Publishers, 1971.

Kordish, Jay. *The Juiceman's Power of Juicing.* New York: Warner Books, 1991.

Lombardi, Susana. *Healthy Living, A Holistic Guide.* We Care Health Ranch Publishers, 1997.

Chapter 9: The Second Principle: Go Organic

There is absolutely no doubt in my mind that your long-term health depends on avoiding potentially dangerous agrichemicals in your food such as pesticides, fungicides, and herbicides. They are toxins. A very important way to do that is to choose organic foods. I've learned about that from many books and monographs. Public service groups—Greenpeace, Mothers and Others, National Organic Directory, and others—are excellent resources for learning more about this topic. Also, the Life Extension Foundation (www.lef.org.) publishes articles in its journal from time to time showing how conventional agriculture has depleted our soil of its nutrient inheritance.

Monograph and newspaper articles

Organic Power: Positive Choices for the Earth and You. Wild Oats Markets, Boulder, Colo., (800) 494-WILD.

Marian Burros. "U.S. imposes standards for organic food labeling," *New York Times,* December 21, 2000.

"Food safety and quality as affected by organic farming." UN Food and Agriculture Organization (FAO) report, July 2000; www.fao.org/organicag/frame2-e.htm

Books

Robbins, John. *The Food Revolution: How Your Diet Can Help Save Your Life and the World.* Berkeley, Calif.: Conari Press, 2001.

Schlosser, Eric. *Fast Food Nation: The Dark Side of the All American Meal.* Boston: Houghton Mifflin, 2001.

Weil, Andrew, and Rosie Daily. *The Healthy Kitchen: Recipes for a Better Body, Life, and Spirit.* New York: Alfred Knopf, 2002.

Scientific article

Organic foods supermarket foods: element levels. *J Appl Nutr* 1993; 45:35–9.

Chapter 10: The Third Principle: Limit or Eliminate Genetically Engineered Foods

There are many excellent articles, books, and Web sites on this subject.

General articles

The commercial cultivation of genetically engineered crops. *Environment* 1999;41:11–21. This is an excellent review article with over 50 references.

Losey JE, Rayor LS, Carter ME. Transgenic pollen harms monarch larvae. *Nature* 1999;399:254.

D. Barboza. "As biotech crops multiply, consumers get little choice." *New York Times,* June 10, 2001. Business Section. Read on the Internet. Describes how more than 100 million acres of the world's most fertile farmland were planted with genetically engineered crops in the year 2000—about twenty-five times as much as just four years earlier.

Books

Anderson, Luke. *Genetic Engineering, Food, and our Environment.* White River Junction, Vt.: Chelsea Green, 1999.

Cummins, Ronnie, and Ben Lilliston. *Genetically Engineered Food.* New York: Marlowe & Company, 2000.

McHughen, Alan. *Pandora's Picnic Basket.* Oxford, England: Oxford University Press, 2000.

Nottingham, Stephen. *Eat Your Genes.* Cape Town, South Africa: University of Cape Town Press, 1998.

Rissler, Jane, and Margaret Mellon. *The Ecological Risks of Engineered Crops*. Cambridge, Mass.: MIT Press, 1996.

Robbins, John. *The Food Revolution*. Berkeley, Calif.: Conari Press, 2001.

Roizen, Michael, and John La Puma. *The RealAge Diet*. New York: HarperCollins, 2001.

Ticciati, Laura, and Robin Ticciati. *Genetically Engineered Foods*. Los Angeles: Keats Publishing, 1998.

Chapter 11: The Fourth Principle: Eat Clean Protein

Many of the same references for the last two chapters apply here as well. Other references include the following:

Monographs

Clean Protein: A Natural Approach to Meats, Poultry, and Seafood. Monograph published by Wild Oats Markets, Boulder Colo., 1998.

Soy Foods. Monograph published by Wild Oats Markets, Boulder Colo., 1998.

Books

Chopra, Deepak, and David Simon. *Grow Younger, Live Longer: 10 Steps to Reverse Aging*. New York: Harmony Books, 2001.

Balch, Phyllis, and James Balch. *Prescription for Nutritional Healing*. New York: Avery, 2000.

Balch, Phyllis, and James Balch. *Prescription For Dietary Wellness*. New York: Avery, 1998.

Medical articles

Goodman MT, Wilkens LR. Association of soy and fiber consumption with the risk of endometrial cancer. *Am J Epidemiol* 1997;146:294–306.

Shu XO, Jin F. Soyfood intake during adolescence and subsequent risk of breast cancer among Chinese women. *Cancer Epidemiol Biomark Prev* 2001; 10:483–88.

Wu AH, Ziegler RG. Tofu and risk of breast cancer in Asian-Americans. *Cancer Epidemiol Biomark Prev* 1996;5:901–6.

Wu AH, Ziegler RG. Soy intake and risk of breast cancer in Asians and Asian Americans. *Am J Clin Nutr* 1998;68:1437S–3S.

Anderson JW, Johnstone BM. Meta-analysis of the effects of soy protein intake on serum lipids. *N Engl J Med* 1995;333:276–82.

Kagawa Y. Eicospolyenoic acids of serum lipids of Japanese islanders with low incidence of cardiovascular diseases. *J Nutr Sci Vitaminol* 1982;28:441–53.

Stroll BA. Essential fatty acids, insulin resistance, and breast cancer risk. *Nutr Cancer* 1998;31:72–7.

See Appendix E, Resources, for additional important Web sites.

Chapter 12: The Fifth Principle: Discover Juicing and Supplements

Most of the ideas about special juices come from years of study and experience. The following have helped shape my thinking: Yogi Bhajan, Dr. Guru Dev Singh Khalsa of Brazil, the late Dr. Paavo Airola, and Dr. Bernard Jensen. I derived many of the juices on my own, but, as mentioned in the text some came from Miraval Life in Balance Resort, where Cari Neff is the executive chef. The folks at Wild Oats Markets on Sunrise in Tucson were also kind enough to share information about juice combinations with me.

The juice book references mentioned in the notes to chapter 1 also apply here.

Journals and newsletters

Life Extension. The Life Extension Foundation monthly journal is very scientific and up to date.

The Health and Healing Newsletter by Julian Whitaker, M.D., has been very useful in supplying authoritative scientific information on vitamin, mineral, and specific nutrient supplementation: www.drwhitaker.com

Nutritional Therapy in Medical Practice: Reference Manual and Study Guide (2001) by Alan Gaby, M.D., provided a wealth of information about the use of vitamins.

Chapter 13: The Sixth Principle: Cook Consciously and Eat Mindfully

Weil, Andrew. *Eating Well for Optimum Health.* New York: Alfred Knopf, 2001.

Ornish, Dean. *Eat More, Weigh Less.* New York: HarperCollins, 1993.

Khalsa, Siri Ved Kaur. *Conscious Cookery.* Los Angeles, Calif.: KRI, 1981.

Bhajan, Yogi. *The Ancient Art of Self-Healing.* Eugene, Ore.: West Anandpur Publishers, 1982.

Chapter 14: The Seventh Principle: Make the Transition

All the preceding books and monographs are useful guides in understanding the background for this chapter. Beyond that, the information came from my own clinical practice. The following books and monographs are very useful as well.

Vegetarian Transition. Monograph produced by Wild Oats Markets, Boulder, Colo., www.wildoats.com

Bhajan, Yogi. *The Ancient Art of Self-Healing.* Eugene, Ore.: West Anandpur Publishers, 1982.

Khalsa, Deva. *Recipes to Purify your Body, Mind and Spirit.* Espanola, N. Mex.: The New Cleanse, 2002, www.thenewcleanse.com

Khalsa, Shakta Kaur. *Kundalini Yoga.* New York: DK Publishing, 2001, 200–15.

Chapter 15: Basic Yoga Nutritional Therapy
Same References as Chapter 13 & 14.

PART TWO
Eat This for That

Books

Neff, Cari. *Conscious Cuisine.* Naperville, Ill.: Sourcebooks, Inc., 2002.

The Life Extension Foundation. *Disease Prevention and Treatment.* Life Extension Media, 2000.

Calbom, Cherie, and Maureen Keane. *Juicing for Life.* New York: Avery, 1992.

Khalsa, Shakta Kaur. *Kundalini Yoga.* New York: Dorling Kindersley Publishing, 2001.

Balch, Phyllis A., and James F. Balch. *Prescription for Dietary Wellness.* New York: Avery, 1992.

Balch, Phyllis A., and James F. Balch. *Prescription for Nutritional Healing.* New York: Avery, 2000.

Chopra, Deepak, and David Simon. *The Chopra Center Herbal Handbook.* New York: Three Rivers Press, 2000.

Bhajan, Yogi. *The Golden Temple Vegetarian Cookbook.* Delhi, India: Ajanta Books International, 1978.

Khalsa, Dharma Singh, and Cameron Stauth. *The Pain Cure.* New York: Warner Books, 1999.

Chapter 16: Addictions

Hoyumpa AM. Mechanisms of vitamin deficiencies in alcoholism. *Alcoholism: Clin Esp Res* 1986;10:573–81.

Free V, Sanders P. The use of ascorbic acid and mineral supplements in the detoxification of narcotic addicts. *J Orthomolecular Psychiatry* 1978;7:264.

Chapter 17: Allergies

Ruskin SL. Sodium ascorbate in the treatment of allergic disturbances. *Am J Dig Dis* 1947;14:302–6.

Johnston CS, et al. Antihistamine effects and complications of supplemental vitamin C. *J Am Diet Assoc* 1992;92:988–9.

Soutar A, et al. Bronchial reactivity and dietary antioxidants. *Thorax* 1997;52:166–70.

Chapter 18: Anti-Aging

Books

Klatz, Ronald M., *Advances in Anti-Aging Medicine*. Vol. 1. Larchmont, NY: Mary Ann Liebert, Inc., 1996.

Klatz, Ronald M., and Robert Goldman. *Anti-Aging Medical Therapeutics*. Vol. II. Del Rey: Health Quest Publications, 1998.

Klatz, Ronald M., and Robert Goldman. *The Science of Anti-Aging Medicine*. Colorado Springs: American Academy of Anti-Aging Medicine, 1996.

Klatz, Ronald, and Robert Goldman. *Stopping the Clock*. New Canaan, Conn.: Keats Publishing, 1996.

Klatz, Ronald M., and Carol Kahn. *Grow Young with HGH*. New York: HarperCollins, 1997.

Schachter-Shalomi, Zalmon, and Ronald S. Miller. *From Age-ing to Sage-ing: A Profound New Vision of Growing Older*. New York: Warner Books, 1995.

Medical articles

Conference report: calorie restriction, exercise, hormone replacement and phytonutrients fight aging. *Life Extension* June 2002;38–46.

Alberg AJ, et al. Serum DHEA and DHEA-S and the subsequent risk of developing colon cancer. *Cancer Epidemiol Biomarkers Prevention* 2000;9:517–21.

Barret-Connor E, et al. Endogenous levels of DHEA-S, but not other sex hormones, are associated with depressed mood in older women: the Rancho Bernardo Study. *J Am Geriatr Soc* 1999;47:685–91.

Ferrari E, et al. Age-related changes of the hypothalamic-pituitary-adrenal axis: pathophysical correlates. *Eur J Endocrinol* 2001;144:319–29.

Reiter WJ, et al. DHEA in the treatment of erectile dysfunction: a prospective, double-blinded, randomized, placebo-controlled study. *Urology* 1999;53:590–4.

Stoll BA. Dietary supplements of DHEA in relation to breast cancer risk. *Eur J Clin Nutr* 1999;53:771–5.

Chapter 19: Attention Deficit Disorder and Attention Deficit Hyperactivity Disorder (ADHD)

Medical articles

Prinz RJ, et al. Dietary correlates of hyperactive behavior in children. *J Consult Clin Psychol* 1980;48:760.

Rapp DJ. Does diet affect hyperactivity? *J Learning Dis* 1978;11:383–9.

Coleman M, et al. A preliminary study of the effect of pyridoxine administration in a subgroup of hyperkinetic children: a double-blind crossover comparison with methylphenidate. *Biol Psychiatry* 1979;14:741.

Brenner A. The effects of megadoses of selected B complex vitamins on children with hyperkinesis: controlled studies with long term followup. *J Learning Dis* 1982;15:258.

Stevens LJ, et al. Essential fatty acid metabolism in boys with attention-deficit hyperactivity disorder. *Am J Clin Nutr* 1995;62:761–8.

Louwman MW, van Dusseldorp M, van de Vijer FJR, et al. Signs of impaired cognitive function in adolescents with marginal cobalamin status. *Am J Clin Nutr* 2000;72:762–69.

Chapter 20: Brain: Age-Associated Memory Impairment (AAMI), Mild Cognitive Impairment (MCI), and Alzeimer's Disease

Medical articles

Fahn S. A pilot trial of high-dose alpha-tocopherol and ascorbate in early Parkinson's disease. *Ann Neurol* 1992;32:S128–32.

Crook T, et al. Effects of phosphatidylserine in Alzheimer's diease. *Psychopharmacol Bull* 1992;28:61–6.

Crook TH, et al. Effects of phosphatidylserine in age-associated memory impairment. *Neurology* 1991;41:644–9.

Sano M, et al. A controlled trial of selegiline, alpha-tocopherol, or both as treatment for Alzheimer's disease. *N Engl J Med* 1997;336:1216–22.

Khalsa DS. Integrated medicine and the prevention and reversal of memory loss. *Altern Ther Health Med* 1998;4:38–43.

Nourhashemi F, Gillette-Guyonnet S, Andrieu S, et al. Alzheimer disease: protective factors. *Am J Clin Nutr* 2002;71:643S–9S.

Chapter 21: Cancer Prevention and Treatment

Medical articles

Black HS, et al. Evidence that a low-fat diet reduces the occurrence of non-melanoma skin cancer. *Int J Cancer* 1995;62:165–9.

Clark LC, et al. Effects of selenium supplementation for cancer prevention in patients with carcinoma of the skin. *JAMA* 1996;276:1957–63.

Clark LC, et al. Decreased incidence of prostate cancer with selenium supplementation: results of a double-blind cancer prevention trial. *Br J Urol* 1998;81:730–4.

Giovannucci E, et al. Intake of carotenoids and retinal in relation to risk of prostate cancer. *J Natl Cancer Inst* 1995;87:1767–76.

Gogos CA, et al. Dietary omega-3 polyunsaturated fatty acids plus vitamin E restore immunodeficiency and prolong survival for severely ill patients with generalized malignancy: a randomized control trial. *Cancer* 1998;82:395–402.

Gonzales NJ, et al. Evaluation of pancreatic proteolytic enzyme treatment of adenocarcinoma of the pancreas, with nutrition and detoxification support. *Nutr Cancer* 1999;33:117–24.

Heimburger DC, Alexander CB, Birch R, et al. Improvement in bronchial squamous metaplasia in smokers treated with folate and vitamin B12. *JAMA* 1988;259:1525–30.

Lamm DL, et al. Megadose vitamins in bladder cancer: a double-blind clinical trial. *J Urol* 1994;151:21–6.

Levy J, et al. Lycopene is a more potent inhibitor of human cancer cell proliferation than either alpha-carotene or beta-carotene. *Nutr Cancer* 1995;24:257–66.

Lichtenstein P. Environmental and heritable factors in the causation of cancer. *N Engl J Med* 2000;343:78–85.

Lissoni P, et al. Modulation of cancer endocrine therapy by melatonin: a phase II study of tamoxifen plus melatonin in metastatic breast cancer patients progressing under tamoxifen alone. *Br J Cancer* 1995;71:854–6.

Lockwood K, et al. Apparent partial remission of breast cancer in "high risk" patients supplemented with nutritional antioxidants, essential fatty acids and coenzyme Q10. *Molec Aspects Med* 1994;15(Suppl):S231–40.

Lockwood K, et al. Progress on therapy of breast cancer with coenzyme Q10 and the regression of metastases. *Biochem Biophys Res Commun* 1995;212:172–7.

The Alpha-Tocopherol, Beta Carotene Cancer Prevention Study Group. The effect of vitamin E and beta carotene on the incidence of lung cancer and other cancers in male smokers. *N Engl J Med* 1994;330:1029–35.

Fairfield K, Fletcher R. Vitamins for chronic disease prevention in adults: scientific review and clinical applications. *JAMA* 2002;287:3116–29.

Monograph

Moving towards a plant-based diet. Monograph published by the American Institute for Cancer Research, Washington, DC, 2000.

Counseling women with respect to lifestyles, life events, and breast cancer risks. Monograph published by the American Cancer Society, Atlanta, Georgia, 1990.

Books

The Life Extension Foundation. *Disease Prevention and Treatment.* Hollywood, Fla.: Life Extension Media, 2000.

Harkness, Richard. *Everything You Need to Know About Reducing Cancer Risk.* Roseville, Calif., Prima Publishing, 2001.

Chapter 22: Children's Health

Medical articles

Iacono G, et al. Intolerance of cow's milk and chronic constipation in children. *N Engl J Med* 1998:339:1100–4.

Chapter 23: Chronic Fatigue

Medical articles

Komaroff AL, et al. Chronic fatigue syndrome: an update. *Annu Rev Med* 1998;49:1–13.

Cunha BA. Beta-carotene stimulation of natural killer cell activity in adult patients with chronic fatigue syndrome. *CFIDS Chronicle Physicians' Forum* 1993;(fall):18.

Howard JM, et al. Magnesium and chronic fatigue syndrome. *Lancet* 1992;340:426.

Chapter 24: Chronic Pain: Arthritis, Backache or Sciatica, Fibromyalgia, and Headache

Medical articles

Leone M, et al. Melatonin versus placebo in the prophylaxis of cluster headache: a double-blind pilot study with parallel groups. *Cephalalgia* 1996;16:494–6.

Paalzow GH. L-dopa induces opposing effects on pain in intact rats: (-)-sulpiride, SCH 23390 or alpha-methyl-DL-tyrosine methylester hydrochloride reveals profound hyperalgesia in large anti-nociceptive doses. *J Pharmacol Exp Ther* 1992;263:470–9.

Peikert A, et al. Prophylaxis of migraine with oral magnesium: results from perspective, multi-center, placebo-controlled and double-blind randomized study. *Cephalalgia* 1996;16:257–63.

Romano TJ, et al. Magnesium deficiency in fibromyalgia syndrome. *J Nutr Med* 1994;4:165–7.

Books

Khalsa, Dharma Singh, and Cameron Stauth. *The Pain Cure.* New York: Warner Books, 1999.

Chapter 25: Cleansing and Detoxification

Books
Bhajan, Yogi. *The Ancient Art of Self-Healing.* Eugene, Ore.: West Anand-pur Publications, 1982.

Chapter 26: Depression

Medical articles
Coppen A, Bailey J. Enhancement of the antidepressant action of fluoxe-tine by folic acid: a randomized, placebo controlled trial. *J Affect Disord* 2000; 60:121–30.

Fairfield K, Fletcher R. Vitamins for chronic disease prevention in adults: scientific review and clinical applications. *JAMA* 2002;287:3116–29.

Stoll AL, et al. Omega-3 fatty acids in bipolar disorder: a preliminary double-blind, placebo-controlled trial. *Arch Gen Psychiatry* 1999;56:407–12.

Monograph
Walsh, W. *Nutrients Help Alleviate Mental Symptoms.* Monograph pub-lished by Well Being, Inc., North Bend, Wash., 2002.

Chapter 27: Diabetes

Medical articles
Friedberg CE, et al. Fish oil and glycemic control in diabetes: a meta-analysis. *Diabetes Care* 1998;21:494–500.

Tutuncu NB, et al. Reversal of defective nerve conduction with vitamin E supplementation in type 2 diabetes: a preliminary study. *Diabetes Care* 1998; 21:1915–18.

Chapter 28: Digestive Health: Gallbladder, Stomach (Acid and Ulcers), Liver, and Colon (Inflammation, Constipation, and Hemorrhoids)

Medical articles
Thornton JR, et al. Diet and gallstones: effects of refined carbohydrate diets on bile cholesterol saturation and bile acid metabolism. *Gut* 1983;24:2.

Hawthorne AB, et al. Treatment of ulcerative colitis with fish oil supple-mentation: a prospective 12 month randomized controlled trial. *Gut* 1992;33: 922–8.

Books
Segala, Melanie, ed. *The Life Extension Foundation's Disease Prevention and Treatment.* Expanded 3rd edition. *Scientific Protocols That Integrate Main-*

stream and Alternative Medicine. Hollywood, Fla.: Life Extension Media, 2000: 201–4.

Monograph

Nichols, Trent W., and Barry W. Ritz. *Naturally Improve Digestive Health: Healing Leaky Gut.* Monograph published by Well Being, Inc., North Bend, Wash.: 2002.

Chapter 29: Heart Disease, Hypertension, and High Cholesterol

Medical articles

Sinatra, Steven. Coenzyme Q10: a vital therapeutic nutrient for the heart with special application in congestive heart failure. *Conn Med* 1997;61: 707–11.

Fairfield K, Fletcher R. Vitamins for chronic disease prevention in adults: scientific review and clinical applications. *JAMA* 2002;287:3116–29.

Chapter 30: HIV and AIDS

Medical articles

Mulkins A, Morse JM, Best A. Complementary therapy use in HIV/AIDS. *Can J Public Health.* 2002 Jul-Aug;93(4):308–12.

Wu JA, Attele AS, Zhang L, Yuan CS. Anti-HIV activity of medicinal herbs: usage and potential development. *Am J Chin Med.* 2001;29(1):69–81. Review.

Chapter 31: Immune Health

Medical articles

Lampe JW. Health effects of vegetables and fruits: assessing mechanisms of action in human experimental studies. *Am J Clin Nutr.* 1999 Sep;70 (3 Suppl):475S–490S. Review.

Craig WJ. Health-promoting properties of common herbs. *Am J Clin Nutr.* 1999 Sep;70(3 Suppl):491S–499S. Review.

Hayashi A, Gillen AC, Lott JR. Effects of daily oral administration of quercetin chalcone and modified citrus pectin. *Altern Med Rev.* 2000 Dec;5(6):546–52.

Amagase H, Petesch BL, Matsuura H, Kasuga S, Itakura Y. Intake of garlic and its bioactive components. *J Nutr.* 2001 Mar;131(3s):955S–62S. Review.

Chapter 32: Kidney Disease

Medical articles

Curhan GC, et al. A prospective study of dietary calcium and other nutrients and the risk of symptomatic kidney stones. *N Engl J Med* 1993;328:833–8.

Hallson PC, et al. Magnesium reduces calcium oxalate crystal formation in human whole urine. *Clin Sci* 1982;62:17.

Seltzer MA, et al. Dietary manipulation with lemonade to treat hypocitraturic calcium nephrolithiasis. *J Urol* 1996;156:907–9.

Chapter 33: Lung Disease: Asthma and Chronic Obstructive Lung Disease, including Emphysema and Bronchitis

Medical articles

Durevil B, Matuszczak Y. Alteration in nutritional status and diaphragm muscle function. *Reprod Nutr Dev* 1998;38:175–80.

Fiaccadori E, et al. Muscle and serum magnesium in pulmonary intensive care unit patients. *Crit Care Med* 1988;16:751–60.

Balansky RB, et al. Protection by N-acetylcysteine of the histopathological and cytogenetical damage produced by exposure of rats to cigarette smoke. *Cancer Lett* 1992;64:123–31.

Books

Segala, Melanie, ed. *The Life Extension Foundation's Disease Prevention and Treatment.* Expanded 3rd edition. *Scientific Protocols That Integrate Mainstream and Alternative Medicine.* Hollywood, Fla.: Life Extension Media; 2000:272–8.

Chapter 34: Men's Health: Impotence and Prostate Problems

Medical articles

Andro M-C, et al. Pygeum africanum extract for the treatment of patients with benign prostatic hyperplasia: a review of 25 years of published experience. *Curr Ther Res* 1995;56:796–817.

Chen J, et al. Effect of oral administration of high-dose nitric oxide donor L-arginine in men with organic erectile dysfunction: results of a double-blind, randomized, placebo-controlled study. *BJU Int* 1999;83:269–73.

Wilt TJ, et al. Saw palmetto extracts for treatment of benign prostatic hyperplasia: a systematic review. *JAMA* 1998;280:1604–9.

Fairfield K, Fletcher R. Vitamins for chronic disease prevention in adults: scientific review and clinical applications. *JAMA* 2002;287:3116–29.

Chapter 35: Skin Disorders: Acne and Aging

Medical articles

Berger, Bernard. Effectiveness of antioxidants (vitamin C and E) with and without sunscreens as topical photoprotectants. *Acta Dermatol Venereol* 1996; 76:264–8.

Michaelsson G, et al. Effects of oral zinc and vitamin A in acne. *Arch Dermatol* 1977;113:31.

Whitaker J. Wound healing: heal faster now. *Dr. Julian Whitaker's Health & Healing, Your Definitive Guide to Alternative Health and Anti-Aging Medicine* 2002;12:5–7.

Traikovich S. Use of topical ascorbic acid and its effects on photodamaged skin topography. *Arch Otolaryngol Head Neck Surg* 1999;125:109–8.

Chapter 36: Spiritual Growth

Bhajan, Yogi. *The Master's Touch.* Los Angeles: Kundalini Research Institute, 1997.

Bhajan, Yogi. The Ancient Art of Self-Healing. Eugene, Ore.: West Anandpur Publishers, 1982.

Chapter 37: Stress and Anxiety

Medical articles

Kelly GS. Nutritional and botanical interventions to assist with the adaptation to stress. *Altern Med Rev.* 1999 Aug;4(4):249-65. Review.

Chapter 38: Thyroid

Medical articles

Olivieri O, et al. Low selenium status in the elderly influences thyroid hormones. *Clin Sci* 1995;89:637–42.

D'Avanzo B, et al. Selected micronutrient intake and thyroid carcinoma risk. *Cancer* 1997;79:2186–92.

Forsythe WA 3rd. Soy protein, thyroid regulation and cholesterol metabolism. *J Nutr* 1995;125 (Suppl):619S–23S.

Mano T, et al. Vitamin E and coenzyme Q concentrations in the thyroid tissues of patients with various thyroid disorders. *Am J Med Sci* 1998;315:230–2.

Chapter 39: Weight Loss

Medical articles

Striffler JS, et al. Chromium improves insulin response to glucose in rats. *Metabolism* 1995;44:1314–20.

Mertz W. Chromium in human nutrition: a review. *J Nutr* 1993;123:626–33.

Blair SN, Nichaman MZ. The public health problem of increasing prevalence rates of obesity and what should be done about it. *Mayo Clinic Proc.* 2000;77:109–13.

Jain M, et al. Tumour characteristics and survival of breast cancer patients in relation to premorbid diet and body size. *Breast Cancer Res Treat.* 1997;42:43–55.

Pi-Sunyer FX. The fattening of America. *JAMA* 1994;272:238–9.

Chapter 40: Women's Health: Fibrocystic Breast Disease, Menopause, Osteoporosis, Premenstrual Syndrome (PMS), and Uterine Fibroids

Medical articles

Albertazzi P, et al. The effect of dietary soy supplementation on hot flushes. *Obstet Gynecol* 1998;91:6–11.

Fairfield K, Fletcher R. Vitamins for chronic disease prevention in adults: scientific review and clinical applications. *JAMA* 2002;287:3116–29.

Facchinetti F, et al. Oral magnesium successfully relieves premenstrual mood changes. *Obstet Gynecol* 1991;78:177–81.

Preisinger E, et al. Nutrition and osteoporosis: an analysis of dietary intake in postmenopausal women. *Wien Klin Wochenschr* 1995;107:418–22.

Choay P, et al. Value of micronutrient supplementals in the prevention of disturbances accompanying the menopause. *Rev Fr Gynecol Obstet* 1990; 85:702–5.

Taffe AM, et al. "Natural" hormone replacement therapy and dietary supplements used in the treatment of menopausal symptoms. *Prim Care Pract* 1998;2:292–302.

Shoff SM, et al. Usual consumption of plant foods containing phytoestrogens and sex hormone levels in postmenopausal women in Wisconsin. *Nutr Cancer* 1998;30:207–12.

Lieberman S. A review of the effectiveness of Cimicifuga racemosa (black cohosh) for the symptoms of menopause. *J Womens Health* 1998;7:525–9.

Nagata C, et al. Association of diet and other lifestyle with onset of menopause in Japanese women. *Maturitas* 1998;29:105–13.

Acknowledgments

Richard Pine, my agent, for making it happen. Judith Curr, Executive Vice President and Publisher of Atria Books for her support. Tracy Behar, for being a fantastically active editor who always makes a book better. Brenda Copeland, for all her kindness, and Wendy Walker for her assistance in the editing process.

Bill Tonelli was instrumental in helping prepare the manuscript.

I'd like to thank my spiritual teacher Siri Singh Sahib Yogi Bhajan for everything he has done for me. His wife, Bibiji, was, as usual, instrumental and an inspiration in developing yoga nutritional therapy concepts into actual recipes. Deva Kaur Khalsa and Dr. Kartar Singh Khalsa of The Cleanse were kind enough to share their recipes as well. Deepest thanks to Sadhana Kaur Khalsa, M.D., and Guru Tej Singh Khalsa for their unwavering support, and to Siri Kartar Kaur Khalsa for her illustrations.

Kirti Kaur Khalsa, my devoted and loving wife, helped me beyond description in the writing, editing, and preparation of this book.

Martin Zamora, my right-hand man, handles the office with dignity and professionalism, for which we are very grateful.

Malcolm Riley, D.D.S., executive director of the Alzheimer's Prevention Foundation International, helped with the preparation of the manuscript.

Thanks to Heidi DeCosmo, sous chef at Miraval, Life in Balance Resort, for helping to review and test the recipes. Also *gracias* to Luz-Elena Shearer, master's degree nutritionist, for her clinical expertise and dedication to our work.

Somers H. White has been my business mentor and coach for close to twenty years. He has made my success possible, and I thank him very much for his insight, advice, and support.

I want to thank Deepak Chopra, M.D., for being such a great role model.

Juan Manuel Mondragon of Mexico City is a man of integrity and vision. For this I salute him.

I would like to also acknowledge the sage Bhai Baldeep Singh Ragi of India and his grand-uncle Bhai Avtar Singh Ragi, a great saint, for their light.

To them and all of you, I offer my thanks. Onward and upward. May all victory be His.

Dharma Singh Khalsa, M.D.
Tucson, Arizona

Index

weight *(cont'd)*
  and supplements, 277; and teas,
    57; and thyroid, 272; and
    vegetables, 276. *See also* obesity
Weight-Loss Tea, 144
wheat, 57, 146–47, 161, 162,
  234, 266
wheat germ, 76, 281
wheat grass, 50, 51, 52, 111, 214
wheatberries, 58, 153–54
whey, 93, 112, 122, 129
whey protein powder, 177–78,
  182–83, 188, 202
white fish, 237
White Turnip Fast, 286
wine, 66
women, 279–86; and aging, 173,
  175; and allergies, 163; and
  detoxification, 70, 71; and diet,
  280, 281, 283, 284, 285; and
  fatigue, 203; and fruit, 40, 281,
  285; and heart disease, 232; and
  herbs, 281–83, 284, 285, 286; and
  juicing, 286; and protein, 104; and
  recipes, 286; and super foods, 53;
  supplements for, 280–82, 283–84,
  285–86; testosterone for, 175; and
  vegetables, 30, 31, 279, 280, 281,
  284, 285; and yoga nutritional
  therapy recipes, 149. *See also*
  fibroids; menopause; osteoporosis;
  premenstrual syndrome

yams, 227
yerba mate tea, 57
yoga, 4, 75, 76, 216
yoga nutritional therapy: ancient
  recipes for, 144–54; and fruit, 40,
  46, 47; overview about, 10,
128–29; principles of, 69; and
  pyramids, 68; recipes for, 140–54;
  resources concerning, 313;
  transition to, 69, 128–39; and
  vegetables, 30, 36
Yoga Nutritional Therapy Energy-
  Plus Drink, 200, 202–3
Yogi Steak—A Vegetable Loaf, 194–95
Yogi Tea: and addictions, 160, 161;
  and cancer, 192; and detoxification,
  74, 76, 77, 78, 80; and fatigue,
  202; and HIV/AIDS, 243; recipe
  for, 138–39; and weight, 278
The Yogis' Weight Loss Monodiet, 278
yogurt: and aging, 264; and brain,
  187–88; and cancer, 195; and
  detoxification, 76, 80, 215; and
  digestion, 229; and GE foods, 92,
  93; and HIV/AIDS, 245, 246; and
  immune system, 249; and juicing,
  112; and protein, 106; and
  pyramids, 64; and skin, 264; and
  spiritual growth, 267; and transition
  to yoga nutritional therapy, 133,
  135; vitamins and minerals in, 123;
  and yoga nutritional therapy
  recipes, 143, 147, 154
Yogurt Curry, 154

zattar, 62, 255
zinc, 115, 117, 122, 123; and aging,
  263; and fruits, 46; and kidneys,
  251; and men's health, 256, 258,
  259, 260; and protein, 100; and
  skin, 262, 263; and thyroid, 273;
  and vegetables, 34
Zinc Boost, 259
zucchini, 80–81, 123, 149–50,
  152, 278